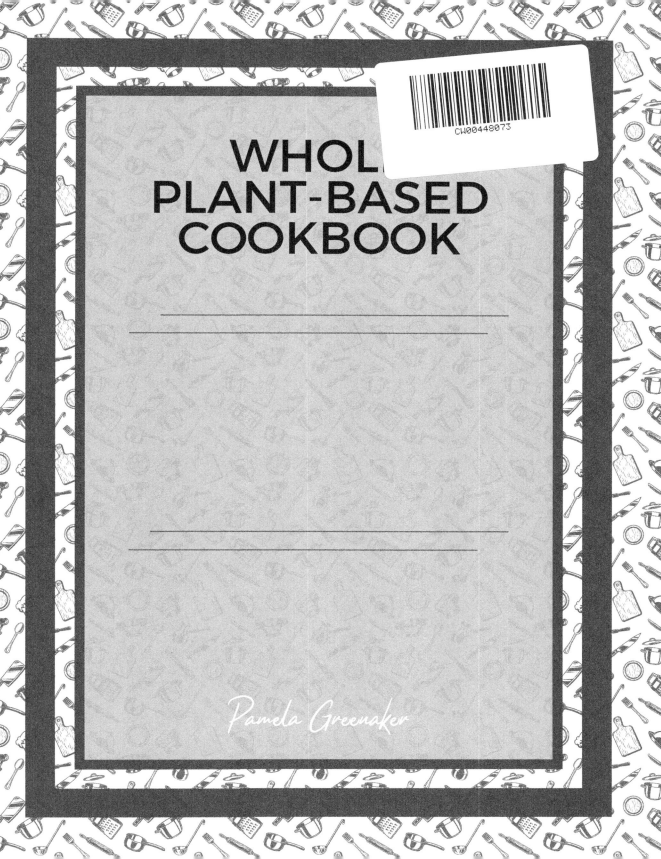

WHOLE PLANT-BASED COOKBOOK

Pamela Greenaker

SOMMARIO

INTRODUCTION

*T*he WFPB (Whole-Foods, Plant-Based) diet is a diet that can be useful for quickly losing excess pounds and improving health, even if, to be precise, more than defining it as a "diet" we should talk about lifestyle.

As for the main features of this approach to nutrition, we remind you that it is fundamentally based on the intake of whole foods and foods of plant origin. The advice given to those who want to follow it includes the fact not to use industrially processed foods, as well as those rich in refined sugars. If possible, the focus should be mainly on foods of non-animal origin. A diet rich in animal protein and processed food weighs us down with chronic inflammation, oxidative stress, and a harmful amount of sugars and saturated fats. Eliminating these stressors has enormous power on our well-being.

The Plant-Based diet is more relaxed on the one hand and more stringent on the other.

More relaxed because it is plant-based, but not exclusively plant-based: products of animal origin are allowed in moderate quantities, but on one condition, namely the excellent quality of the food itself and its certified origin. For example, eggs can be consumed occasionally but only if very fresh, possibly at zero km, from free-range farms where the hens are not exploited but can live outdoors without constraints. The WFPB diet also takes into account the intake of good fat sources, such as: avocado, extra virgin olive oil, coconut oil.

The plant based diet can have a lot of different connotations along with it. Sometimes having a strong misconception can be a roadblock, if you let it color your beliefs and choices. You may agree, or think that it is impossible to get the proper nutrients on a plant based diet. Many people also believe that eating this way must be super expensive. You will find your own path and beliefs as you learn to experiment more.

plant based kitchen

TRUE HEALTHY SIMPLE

CHAPTER 1: THE ADVANTAGES OF THE WHOLE PLANT BASED DIET

Here are some of the many benefits of a WFPB diet:

1. weight control:

It is easy to lose weight and keep fit by eating whole vegetables, because they are very filling (thanks to a low calorie density and the presence of many fibers).

Since you are completely getting rid of sugar alongside any junk foods! The Whole Foods Diet will have a huge impact eventually when it comes to trimming down your fat. Through Whole Foods Diet, you are promoting your mind to pay more attention to the food that you are eating, thus eliminating more fatty foods from your list, which will, in turn, cause your body to eventually lose weight and attain the physique that you have been dreaming of! If you just do a little research, you are bound to find thousands of stories of man and women successfully losing their weight through Whole Foods diet.

2. saving money:

you can save hundreds of dollars a year, in fact the cost of ingredients and raw materials, in plant-based diets, can be more than 30% less than traditional ones.

3. increased energy:

Many people report better sleep, more energy and a high sports performance: the latter because the complex carbohydrates of whole food release their energy very gradually.

Furthermore, vegetable nutrition improves blood circulation and oxygenation.

4. health and longevity: unrefined vegetables have very little saturated fat and cholesterol, are rich in fiber, vitamins, minerals and are characterized by the presence of antioxidants that play a crucial role in slowing the progression of Alzheimer's disease

Several chronic diseases can be avoided, stopped or treated. Among them are diseases of the heart, respiratory system and diabetes.

5. The risk of having a heart attack, stroke or developing various types of cancer can

also be dramatically reduced. In general, inflammation levels in the body are lowered and the immune system is strengthened.

6. The prevention and treatment of diseases, or degenerative states, can give us a life that is not only long, but full of vitality. Also useful against cognitive decline - plant-based foods are characterized by the presence of antioxidants that play a crucial role in slowing the progression of Alzheimer's disease

7. safeguarding the planet and animals: compared to animal husbandry, growing plant foods usually has a much smaller impact on the environment.

8) Sugars, fats and dairy products (especially cheese) are very addicting, comparable to drugs: it is really difficult to change, but you can free yourself.

The gut microbiota, accustomed to animal and industrial food, makes us want the "wrong" things, but luckily this also works the other way around once we get used to healthy food.

A plant-based diet helps improve your gut health. Items sourced from plants are full of rich fiber, and this improves digestion. Fiber will add bulk to stool and regulate the entire digestive process.

As plants are rich in minerals and vitamins, they are great energy boosters. You will find them full of phytonutrients, antioxidants, and healthy protein and fat. All these are good for both the body and the brain. Plant-sourced items are easier to digest, which helps the body by giving it some extra energy.

9. Reduction in the risk of cancers

Three main studies were ran over large groups of dieters that focused on the plant foods over a period. The results showed against those that consumed excess portions of animal and processed food were as follows: - The greater portion that focused on solely plant-based foods had lesser risks in having gastrointestinal and colorectal cancers.

- The other groups that merged the plant-based diet with the lacto-ovo vegetarian diet and pescatarian diet experienced the same results but with higher chances of getting these cancers.

Therefore, this proves that sticking to a whole-foods plant-based diet keeps you a safer from cancers.

10. Prevention of Diabetes

Plant-based foods are excellent at reducing high blood sugars. Many studies comparing the vegetarian and vegan diet to a regular meat filled diet, proved that dieting with more plant foods reduced the risk of diabetes by 50%.

It goes to say that eliminating processed and animal foods from your diet only makes this result read better for you.

11. Improved skin, nails, and hair condition

Let's start with one of the most unexpected benefits first! Once you start to cut down the unhealthy foods from your body, the condition of your skin and nails will start to improve.

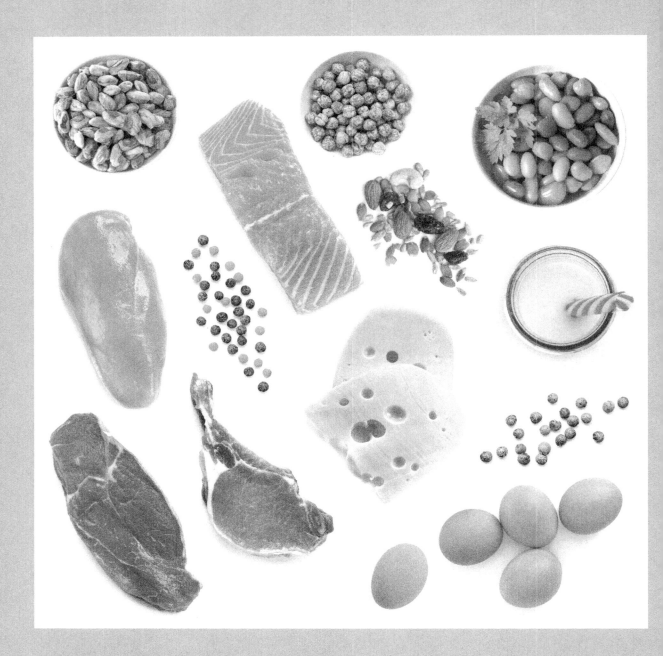

CHAPTER 2: FIRST STEPS

Even if you can gradually approach an increasingly plant-based diet, there is also a good reason to start at 100% right from the start.

Much depends on your personality: whether you find it easier to make a gradual change or whether a radical approach is easier.

A strong motivation is that, the sooner you start giving your body only the best nourishment, the sooner you can notice positive changes: the changes will be encouraging and will help you move forward even before you get used to them.

Any sensations of bloating and bloating, even for weeks, are usually only transient.

In the transition phase, it is possible to feel the effects of body detoxification in the form of a headache or fatigue. But this usually passes within a few days and the positive effects set in.

Food is strongly rooted in the culture, traditions, beliefs and rituals of our families and friends. In addition to habit, there is also social pressure. If you change your course, others sometimes feel challenged and may want to convince you that theirs is the right choice.

Our sense of taste has to get used to. At first, healthy food may not seem very tasty, but once we change our habits we can develop a different sensitivity and fully enjoy the flavors.

Frequent questions

Are you getting enough protein?

Yes: if you eat enough calories and your diet is varied with all plant food groups included, it is automatic to get enough protein. Legumes and grains are the most famous, but other foods also contain essential amino acids in varying quantities. For example, flax seeds and hemp are also excellent sources of protein, but broccoli also has a lot to offer (especially in relation to low calories).

Is it okay at any stage of life?

Yes, a plant-based diet is fine for children, pregnant or breastfeeding women, athletes and the elderly, it is only necessary to consider that for small children you need to limit the amount of fiber a little and increase the amount of fiber a little. fat than the adult.

What are the disadvantages of a WFPB diet?

You have to find the motivation to radically change what you eat. Any significant change requires some commitment and there are so many benefits that can motivate you. You have to learn how to prepare compatible dishes at home and, since at most restaurants there are vegan solutions, it can be a little more difficult to eat out: but even at the restaurant you can find satisfying compromises, such as a whole-meal pizza with vegetables, or potatoes. baked with a plate of grilled vegetables.

When you eat only vegetables, it is important to supplement vitamin B12 with a supplement. Few people know that the vitamin B12 contained in meat nowadays is only present because animals are also given supplements of this vitamin, therefore, better avoid the harmful effects of meat (including all antibiotics given) and take a good supplement ourselves

To determine what your body is doing, start by taking a close look at your current diet. Keep a food journal for a week, to allow yourself to see what it is that your body consumes on a daily basis. Your journal should include:

Food eaten at all meals, including all condiments such as butter, sour cream, dressing, syrup, etc...

All snacks

All beverages

Don't overlook anything that you consume; it all counts towards your calorie count as well as your nutritional values. When you are conscious about what you are eating, you might realize that your diet is not as healthy as you once thought. Then you can determine how to start making changes.

The Foods to Eat

If you slowly start to replace your current diet with plant based foods that are direct from the source, you will begin to give your body what it craves. There are significantly fewer calories in a plate full of healthy vegetables, rather than a big, juicy steak that was cooked in butter with a loaded baked potato on the side. Does this mean that you have to give up that steak dinner forever? No, it simply means that you need to learn to modify your food choices. Once in a while it is okay to give into your cravings for a meat dinner; you just need to make different choices by cooking without butter or oils, avoid over cooking your vegetables to retain their nutrients and their taste and eliminating fattening condiments.

Now that I talk of plant-focused foods, let's count the many options that you can enjoy.

● Fruits

All fruits are permitted on the plant-based diet and they can be enjoyed either fresh, frozen, or sun-dried. Eat the wide range of citrus fruits, berries, grapes, apples, melons, bananas, peaches, apricots, avocado, kiwi fruits, **etc.**

● Vegetables

A healthful plant-based sits in a wide range of vegetables. All vegetables are welcomed on the diet both above the ground and under the ground vegetables. Meanwhile, vegetables provide a wide range of vitamins and minerals.

Enjoy spinach, kale, mustard greens, collard greens, broccoli, cauliflower, asparagus, green beans, eggplants, carrots, tomatoes, bell peppers, zucchinis, beetroot, parsnips, turnips, potatoes, **etc.**

● Legumes

Legumes are an excellent source for plant-based protein and fiber. Fiber is one nutrient that many people lack; hence, it is necessary to consume foods like legumes often to enrich the body with enough fiber.

Eat the wide range of beans, chickpeas, lentils, peas, **etc.**

● Nuts and Nut Butters

Nuts are an essential source of selenium, vitamin E, and plant-based protein. They are excellent additions to smoothies, puddings, desserts, and snacks.

Crunch on almonds, pecans, walnuts, macadamia nuts, hazelnuts, pistachios, cashew nuts, peanuts, brazil, **etc.**

● Seeds

Incorporate seeds into soups, snacks, smoothies, desserts, **etc.** They are rich in calcium, Vitamin E, and are a good source of healthy fats.

Consume flaxseeds, pepitas (pumpkin seeds), sunflower seeds, chia seeds, hemp seeds, sesame seeds, **etc.**

● Healthy Oils and Fats

Fats do not have to come from animal sources only. Some plant foods equally provide excellent fats for frying, searing, baking, and act as replacement for most dairy products. Meanwhile, they are rich in omega-3 fatty acids.

Use olive oil, avocados, canola oil, walnuts, peanuts, hemp seeds, flaxseeds, chia seeds, cashew nuts, coconut oil, **etc.**

● Plant-Based Milk, Cream, and Cheeses
Going plant-based doesn't mean starving

yourself off creamy, milky, cheesy foods. You can enjoy plant-based alternatives of pasta alfredo, cheesecakes, **etc.**

Enjoy almond milk, soy milk, coconut milk, coconut cream, rice milk, cashew milk, cashew cream, hemp milk, oats milk, **etc.**

• Plant-Based Meats

Also, enrich your foods with meats options made from plant sources like soymilk and whole grains.

Eat tofu, tempeh, seitan, **etc.**

• Spices, Herbs, and Condiments Nothing beats the preparation of foods than the aroma that exudes while cooking. Therefore, all ranges of homemade spices, herbs, and condiments are welcomed.

Use basil, parsley, rosemary, oregano, thyme, sage, marjoram, turmeric, curry, black pepper, salt, salsa, soy sauce, nutritional yeast, vinegar, homemade BBQ sauce, homemade plant-based mayonnaise, **etc.**

• Beverages

Coffee, sparking water, tea, smoothies, **etc.** are fine to drink.

Foods to Minimize

While healthy animal foods can, at times, be included in such kinds of a diet; you should keep at a minimum such products in all plant-based diets. They include:

• Seafood

• Beef

• Pork

• Mutton

• Game meats

• Poultry products

• Eggs

• Dairy products

This kind of diet is one way of eating healthy, elevating the status of different plant-based diets on the forefront, while cutting down on unhealthy meals, including added sugars and refined grains.

Plant-based diets have been linked directly to a myriad of health benefits, including a reduction in the risk of heart disease, certain types of cancers, obesity, diabetes, and a decline in our cognitive abilities. Additionally, it is worthy to transition to a more plant-based diet for our good. Irrespective of the kinds of whole-foods, a plant-based diet, which you have chosen, one thing for sure is that you are bound to lead a healthy life in the end.

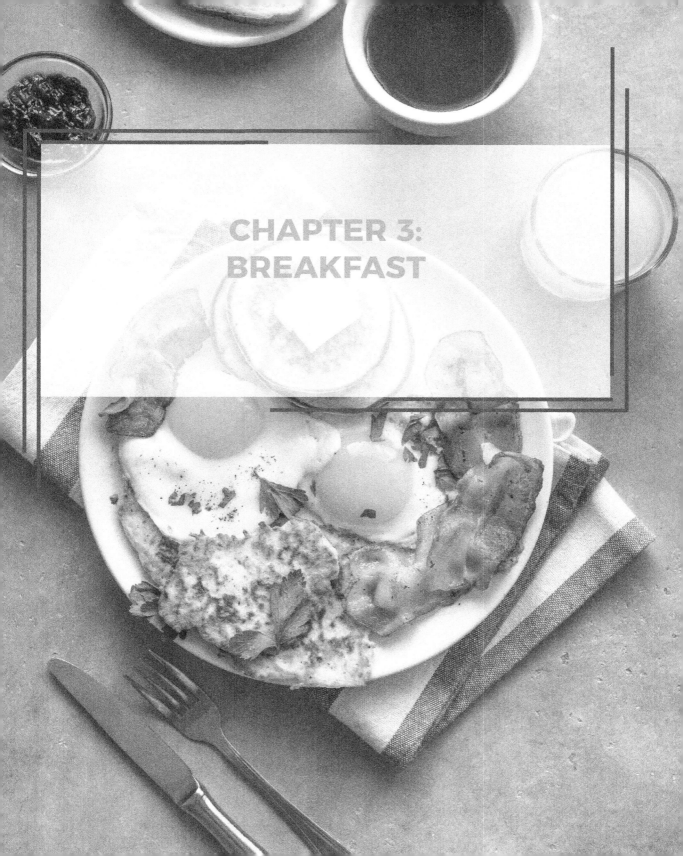

CHAPTER 3: BREAKFAST

Preparation Time: 10 minutes
Cooking Time: 30 minutes
Servings: 5

1. Cranberry Muffins

INGREDIENTS:

- 1 cup almond flour
- ½ cup stevia
- 1 teaspoon baking soda
- ½ teaspoon nutmeg, ground
- ¼ cup natural apple juice
- ¼ cup avocado oil
- 2 tablespoons flaxseed mixed with 3 tablespoons water
- 1 cup fresh cranberries
- 2 teaspoons ginger, grated
- ¼ cup pecans, chopped
- Cooking spray

DIRECTIONS:

1. In a large bowl, combine the flour with stevia, baking soda and the other ingredients except the cooking spray and stir well.
2. Grease a muffin tray with cooking spray, divide the muffin mix, introduce in the oven and cook at 375 degrees F for 30 minutes.
3. Divide the muffins between plates and serve for breakfast.

Nutrition: *calories 212, fat 3.2, fiber 6.1, carbs 14, protein 6*

Preparation Time: 10 minutes
Cooking Time: 25 minutes
Servings: 4

2. Pineapple Oatmeal

INGREDIENTS:

- 2 cups old-fashioned oats
- 2 cups pineapple, cubed
- 1 tablespoon stevia
- 2 cups almond milk
- 2 tablespoons flaxmeal mixed with 3 tablespoons water
- 2 teaspoons almond extract

DIRECTIONS:

1. In a large bowl mix the oats with pineapple and the other ingredients, stir and divide into 4 ramekins
2. Introduce in the oven and cook at 400 degrees F for 25 minutes.
3. Serve for breakfast.

Nutrition: *calories 201, fat 4.4, fiber 4, carbs 5.4, protein 6*

Preparation Time: 30 minutes
Cooking Time: 4 minutes
Servings: 4

3. Miso Oat Porridge

INGREDIENTS:

- 1 cup Steel cut oats
- 1 teaspoon miso paste
- 1 tablespoon tahini
- ½ avocado, peeled
- ½ teaspoon nutritional yeast
- 2 cups almond milk
- 1 ½ teaspoon chives, chopped

DIRECTIONS:

1. Mix up together almond milk, nutritional yeast, and tahini.
2. Then pour the liquid in the instant pot bowl.
3. Add steel cut oats and stir gently. Close the lid.
4. Cool the oats on High Pressure for 4 minutes.
5. Then allow natural pressure release for 25 minutes.
6. Meanwhile, mash the avocado well.
7. Add miso paste and chives. Stir until smooth.
8. Transfer the cooked oats in the bowl and add avocado mash. Stir carefully.

Nutrition: *calories 394, fat 36.4, fiber 5.9, carbs 16.9, protein 5.7*

Preparation Time: 10 minutes
Cooking Time: 30 minutes
Servings: 4

4. Mushroom Patties

INGREDIENTS:

- 1 yellow onion, minced
- 1/2 tsp. cumin
- 15 oz. canned pinto beans, drained
- 3/4 cup mushrooms, chopped
- 1 tsp. parsley leaves, chopped
- Salt and black pepper, to taste
- 1 tbsp. canola oil
- 1 garlic clove, minced
- 3 green onion, minced
- A drizzle olive oil, for frying

DIRECTION

1. Set your instant pot on Sauté mode. Add canola oil and heat it up.
2. Add garlic and yellow onion. Stir and cook for 5 minutes.
3. Add mushroom, green onions, salt, pepper and cumin.
4. Stir, cover and cook on Low for 5 minutes.
5. Release pressure quickly.
6. Transfer mushrooms mix to a bowl and leave it aside to cool down.
7. Put the beans in your food processor, blend a few times and add them to mushroom mix.
8. Add more salt and pepper to the taste and parsley. Stir very well.
9. Shape the patties. Heat up a pan with some olive oil over medium high heat.
10. Add burgers and cook for 3 minutes on each side. Serve and enjoy!

Nutrition: *calories 120, fat 28g, fiber 1g, carbs 8g, protein 23g*

Preparation Time: 10 minutes
Cooking Time: 15 minutes
Servings: 4

5. Peaches Oatmeal

INGREDIENTS:

- 1 tsp. vanilla extract
- 2 tbsp. flax meal
- 4 cups water
- 1 peach, chopped
- 2 cups rolled oats
- 1/2 almonds, chopped

DIRECTION

1. In your instant pot, mix water with peach, oats, vanilla extract, flax meal and almonds.
2. Stir, cover and cook on High for 3 minutes.
3. Stir again and divide into bowls. Serve and enjoy!

Nutrition: *calories 143, fat 5.9, fiber 4.2, carbs 9, protein*

Preparation Time: 10 minutes
Cooking Time: 12 minutes
Servings: 4

6. Poached Figs

INGREDIENTS:

- 1/2 cup pine nuts
- 1 cup red wine
- 1 pound figs
- Stevia, to taste

DIRECTION

1. Put the wine in your instant pot. Add stevia to taste and stir well.
2. Add steamer basket and put the figs inside.
3. Cover and cook on Low for 3 minutes.
4. Divide figs into bowls. Drizzle wine over them.
5. Sprinkle pine nuts at the end. Serve and enjoy!

Nutrition: *Calories 393 kcal Fats 17. 1g Carbs 31. 9g Protein 27. 8g*

Preparation Time: 10 minutes
Cooking Time: 20 minutes
Servings: 4

7. Quinoa and Veggie Mix

INGREDIENTS:

- Zest from 1/2 lemon, grated
- 4 garlic cloves, minced
- A pinch salt and black pepper
- 1 cup red quinoa
- 10 cherry tomatoes, halved
- 1 yellow onion, chopped
- 3 tbsp. olive oil
- 2 small carrots, shredded
- 2 cups button mushrooms, sliced
- 2 tbsp. lemon juice
- 1 cup veggie stock
- 1 tbsp. parsley, chopped

DIRECTION

1. Set your instant pot on Sauté mode. Add oil and heat it up.
2. Add carrot and onion. Stir and cook for 2 minutes.
3. Add mushrooms. Stir and cook for 4 minutes more.
4. Add lemon zest, stock, salt, pepper, quinoa and cherry tomatoes.
5. Stir, cover and cook on High for 10 minutes.
6. Add parsley, toss a bit and divide into bowls. Serve and enjoy!

Nutrition: *Calories 519 kcal Fats 13. 4g Carbs 87. 5g Protein 19. 6g*

Preparation Time: 10 minutes
Cooking Time: 23 minutes
Servings: 4

8. Raspberry Curd

INGREDIENTS:

- Stevia, to taste
- 12 oz. raspberries
- 2 tbsp. lemon juice
- 2 tbsp. vegetable oil
- 2 tbsp. flax meal, mixed with 4 tbsp. water

DIRECTION

1. In your instant pot, mix raspberries with stevia to taste, oil, lemon juice and flax meal.
2. Stir, cover and cook on High for 2 minutes.
3. Stir well and divide into cups. Serve and enjoy!

Nutrition: *calories 350, fat 28g, fiber 1g, carbs 8g, protein 22g*

Preparation Time: 20 minutes
Cooking Time: 8 minutes
Servings: 4

9. Rice Pudding

INGREDIENTS:

- 1 ½ cup of rice
- 3 cups of rice milk
- 1 tablespoon all-purpose flour
- 2 tablespoon sugar
- ¼ teaspoon turmeric
- 1 teaspoon vanilla extract

DIRECTIONS:

1. In the mixing bowl combine together ½ cup of rice milk and all-purpose flour.
2. Add sugar, turmeric, and vanilla extract.
3. Then pour it in the instant pot bowl.
4. Add rice, sugar, and remaining rice milk. Stir gently.
5. Close the lid and set the Manual mode (High pressure).
6. Cook the rice pudding for 8 minutes.
7. Then allow natural pressure release for 20 minutes.
8. Open the lid and stir the rice pudding – it should have a soft but thick texture.

Nutrition: *calories 376, fat 2, fiber 1, carbs 81.8, protein 5.5*

Preparation Time: 8 minutes
Cooking Time: 15 minutes
Servings: 5

10. Rice with Maple Syrup

INGREDIENTS:

- 1 cup of rice
- 2 cups almond milk
- 1 teaspoon vanilla extract
- ¼ cup maple syrup
- 1 teaspoon almond butter

DIRECTIONS:

1. Place rice in the instant pot.
2. Add almond milk and vanilla extract. Stir gently and close the lid.
3. Set the "Rice" mode and cook rice for 15 minutes.
4. Then add almond butter and maple syrup. Stir it.

Nutrition: *calories 419, fat 25, fiber 2.9, carbs 46.2, protein 5.5*

Preparation Time: 10 minutes
Cooking Time: 30 minutes
Servings: 4

11. Strawberry Compote

DIRECTION

In your instant pot, mix strawberries with stevia and leave aside for 10 minutes.

Add orange juice, stir, cover and cook on High for 1 minute.

Divide into small serving cups. Serve and enjoy!

Nutrition: *calories 143, fat 5.9, fiber 4.2, carbs 9, protein*

INGREDIENTS:

* 1 oz. orange juice
* 6 tbsp. stevia
* 1 pound strawberries, halved

Preparation Time: 10 minutes
Cooking Time: 15 minutes
Servings: 4

12. Turnip Dish

INGREDIENTS:

* 1 tbsp. olive oil
* 1 tsp. lemon juice
* 1 cup water
* 2 turnips, peeled and sliced
* 3 carrots, sliced
* 1 small onion, chopped
* 1 tsp. cumin, ground
* Salt and black pepper, to taste

DIRECTION

1. Set your instant pot on Sauté mode. Add oil and heat it up.
2. Add onion, stir and cook for 3 minutes.
3. Add turnips, carrots, cumin, lemon juice, salt, pepper and water.
4. Stir, cover and cook on High for 7 minutes.
5. Divide everything amongst plates. Serve and enjoy!

Nutrition: *calories 127, fat 3.3, fiber 2.8, carbs 22.5, protein 3.2*

Preparation Time: 5 minutes
Cooking Time: 1 hour & 15 minutes
Servings: 4

13. Spiced Sorghum & Berries

INGREDIENTS:

- 1 cup whole-grain sorghum
- 1 teaspoon ground cinnamon
- 1 teaspoon Chinese five-spice powder
- 3 cups water, plus more as needed
- 1 cup unsweetened nondairy milk
- 1 teaspoon vanilla extract
- 2 tablespoons pure maple syrup
- 1 tablespoon chia seeds
- ¼ cup sliced almonds
- 2 cups fresh raspberries, divided

DIRECTIONS:

1. Stir together the sorghum, cinnamon, five-spice powder, and water in a large pot over medium-high heat. Boil the water, cover the pot, and reduce the heat to medium-low.
2. Cook for 1 hour, or until the sorghum is soft and chewy. If the sorghum grains are still hard, add another water cup and cook for 15 minutes more.
3. In a glass measuring cup, whisk together the milk, vanilla, and maple syrup to blend. Add the mixture to the sorghum, along with the chia seeds, almonds, and 1 cup of raspberries.
4. Gently stir to combine. Serve topped with the remaining 1 cup of fresh raspberries.

Nutrition: *Calories: 289, Fat: 8g, Protein: 9g, Carbohydrates: 52g*

Preparation Time: 1 hour & 15 minutes
Cooking Time: 0 minutes
Servings: 4

14. Raw Cinnamon-Apple & Nut Bowl

INGREDIENTS:

- 1 green apple, halved, seeded, and cored
- 3 Honeycrisp apples, halved, seeded, and cored
- 1 teaspoon freshly squeezed lemon juice
- 5 pitted Medjool dates
- ½ teaspoon ground cinnamon
- Pinch ground nutmeg
- 2 tablespoons chia seeds, plus more for serving (optional)
- 1 tablespoon hemp seeds
- ¼ cup chopped walnuts
- Nut butter, for serving (optional)

DIRECTIONS:

1. Finely dice half the green apple and 1 Honeycrisp apple. Put in an airtight container with the lemon juice while you work on the next steps.
2. Coarsely chop the remaining apples and the dates. Transfer to a food processor and add the cinnamon and nutmeg. Pulse several times to combine, then process for 2 to 3 minutes to puree.
3. Stir the puree into the reserved diced apples. Stir in the chia seeds (if using), hemp seeds, and walnuts. Refrigerate for at least 1 hour before serving.
4. Serve as is or top with additional chia seeds and nut butter (if using).

Nutrition: *Calories: 274, Fat: 8g, Protein: 4g, Carbohydrates: 52g*

Preparation Time: 5 minutes
Cooking Time: 10 minutes
Servings: 2

15. Peanut Butter & Cacao Breakfast Quinoa

INGREDIENTS:

- 2/3 cup quinoa flakes
- 1 cup unsweetened nondairy milk, plus more for serving
- 1 cup of water
- ¼ cup raw cacao powder
- 2 tablespoons natural creamy peanut butter
- ¼ teaspoon ground cinnamon
- 2 bananas, mashed
- Fresh berries of choice for serving
- Chopped nuts of choice for serving

DIRECTIONS:

1. In a 6-quart pot over medium-high heat, stir together the quinoa flakes, milk, water, cacao powder, peanut butter, and cinnamon.
2. Cook, stirring, until the batter begins to simmer. Turn the heat to medium-low and cook for 3 to 5 minutes, stirring frequently.
3. Stir in the bananas and cook until hot. Serve topped with fresh berries, nuts, and a splash of milk.

Nutrition: *Calories: 471, Fat: 16g Protein: 18g, Carbohydrates: 69g*

Preparation Time: 15 minutes
Cooking Time: 15 minutes
Servings: 4

16. Cauliflower Scramble

INGREDIENTS:

- 1 yellow onion, diced
- 3 garlic cloves, minced
- 1 green bell pepper, seeded & coarsely chopped
- 1 red bell pepper, seeded & coarsely chopped
- 1 tablespoon water, plus more as needed
- 1 large cauliflower head, cored, florets coarsely chopped to about ½-inch dice
- 1 teaspoon ground turmeric
- ¼ cup nutritional yeast
- ¼ teaspoon ground nutmeg
- ¼ teaspoon cayenne pepper
- ¼ teaspoon freshly ground black pepper
- 1 tablespoon coconut aminos
- 1 (15-ounce) can chickpeas, drained and rinsed

DIRECTIONS:

1. Combine the onion, garlic, and green and red bell peppers in a large nonstick skillet over medium heat.
2. Cook for 2 to 3 minutes, stirring, until the onion is translucent but not browned. Add the water, 1 tablespoon at a time, to avoid sticking or burning, as needed.
3. Add the cauliflower and toss to combine. Cover the skillet and cook within 5 to 6 minutes, or until the cauliflower is fork-tender.
4. In a small bowl, stir together the turmeric, nutritional yeast, nutmeg, cayenne pepper, and black pepper. Set aside.
5. Evenly sprinkle the coconut aminos over the cauliflower mixture and stir to combine. Stir in the spice mixture. Mix in the chickpeas, then cook, uncovered, for 5 minutes to warm.

Nutrition: *Calories: 243, Fat: 3g Protein: 18g, Carbohydrates: 40g*

Preparation Time: 15 minutes
Cooking Time: 25 minutes
Servings: 4

17. Veggie Breakfast Hash

INGREDIENTS:

- 1 tablespoon dried thyme
- 2 rosemary sprigs, leaves removed, and minced
- 1 teaspoon Hungarian paprika
- ½ teaspoon freshly ground black pepper
- 2 large sweet potatoes, cut into ½-inch cubes
- 2 parsnips, cut into ½-inch cubes
- 1 rutabaga, cut into ½-inch cubes
- 2 Yukon Gold potatoes, cut into ½-inch cubes
- 4 large carrots, cut into ½-inch cubes
- 1 large onion, diced
- 3 garlic cloves, minced
- 1 (15-ounce) can of red kidney beans, drained and rinsed
- 1 (15-ounce) can chickpeas, drained and rinsed

DIRECTIONS:

1. Preheat the oven to 375°F. Line a sheet pan with parchment paper. Mix the thyme, rosemary, paprika, and pepper in a small bowl. Set aside.
2. Boil your large pot of water over high heat. Add the sweet potatoes, parsnips, rutabaga, Yukon Gold potatoes, and carrots. Parboil for 2 minutes. Drain well but don't rinse.
3. Transfer to a large bowl. Put the thyme batter and toss to coat. Spread the parboiled vegetables on the prepared sheet pan and sprinkle with the onion and garlic.
4. Bake within 20 minutes, or until the vegetables are fork-tender. In a medium bowl, stir together the kidney beans and chickpeas. Serve with the cooked vegetable hash.

Nutrition: *Calories: 458, Fat: 3g Protein: 17g, Carbohydrates: 94g*

Preparation Time: 5 minutes
Cooking Time: 0 minute
Serving: 1

18. Breakfast in Bangkok

INGREDIENTS

- 2 cucumbers
- 1 peeled gala apple, quartered
- 1/4 cup coconut milk
- 1/4 tbsp fresh ginger root, grated

DIRECTIONS:

1. Press cucumbers and apples though a juicer into a large glass. Stir in coconut milk then garnish with ginger root.

Nutrition: *calories 415, fat 35, fiber 2, carbs 8, protein 20*

Preparation Time: 5 minutes
Cooking Time: 15 minutes
Serving: 2

19. Chocolate and Banana Oatmeal

INGREDIENTS:

- 1 small banana, sliced
- 1 cup rolled oats, old-fashioned
- 1/4 teaspoon salt
- 2 tablespoons chocolate-hazelnut spread
- 2 cups of water

DIRECTIONS:

1. Take a small saucepan, place it over medium-high heat, pour in water, stir in salt, and bring it to a boil.
2. Then add oats, stir until mixed, switch heat to medium level, and cook for 5 minutes or more until the oats have absorbed all the cooking liquid.
3. When done, remove the pan from heat, let the oat stand for 3 minutes and then fluff with a fork. Top oats with banana and chocolate-hazelnut spread and then serve.

Nutrition: *Calories: 190, Carbs: 34g, Fat: 6g, Protein: 4g*

Preparation Time: 10 minutes
Cooking Time: 30 minutes
Serving: 4

20. French Toast with Berry Compote

INGREDIENTS:

For French Toast:
- 4 bread slices, whole-grain, each about 3/4-inch thick
- 1/2 cup chickpea liquid or aquafaba
- 1/4 cup almond flour
- 1/4 teaspoon salt
- 1/8 teaspoon ground cinnamon
- 1/4 tablespoon orange zest
- 1 tablespoon maple syrup
- 3/4 cup almond milk, unsweetened

For Berry Compote:
- 1/2 teaspoon maple syrup
- 1/2 cup frozen blueberries, thawed
- 1/4 cup applesauce

DIRECTIONS:

1. Switch on the oven, then set it to 400 degrees F and let it preheat.
2. Meanwhile, take a medium bowl, add flour in it, cinnamon, salt, maple syrup, and aquafaba and whisk until smooth.
3. Transfer this mixture to a shallow dish, then add orange zest and stir until mixed. Take a skillet pan, place it over medium-low heat, and wait until it gets hot.
4. Then dip or soak each slice of bread into the prepared mixture, let soak for a few seconds, then turn the slice and continue soaking for some more seconds.
5. Transfer bread slice into the heated skillet pan and then cook for 3 minutes per side until golden brown. Transfer toast to a plate and repeat with the remaining bread slices.
6. Take a baking sheet, place a wire rack on it, arrange prepared toast on it, and bake for 10 minutes until crispy.
7. Meanwhile, prepare the berry compote and for this, place berries in a food processor, add maple syrup and apple sauce, and then pulse for 2 minutes until smooth.
8. When done, top the French toast with berry compote and then serve.

Nutrition: *Calories: 440, Carbs: 55g, Fat: 21g, Protein: 10g*

Preparation Time: 10 minutes
Cooking Time: 20 minutes
Serving: 4

21. Chocolate Chip and Coconut Pancakes

INGREDIENTS:

- 2 bananas, sliced
- ¾ cup buckwheat flour
- 1 tablespoon coconut flakes, unsweetened
- 2 tablespoons rolled oats, old-fashioned
- 1/8 teaspoon sea salt
- 1/2 tablespoon baking powder
- 1/3 cup mini chocolate chips, grain-sweetened
- 1/4 cup maple syrup
- 1 teaspoon vanilla extract, unsweetened
- 1/2 tablespoon flaxseeds
- 1/4 cup of water
- 1/2 cup applesauce, unsweetened
- 1 cup almond milk, unsweetened

DIRECTIONS:

1. Take a small saucepan, place it over medium heat, add flaxseeds, pour in water, stir until mixed and cook for 3 minutes or until sticky mixture comes together.
2. Then immediately strain the flaxseed mixture into a cup, discard the seeds, and set aside until required.
3. Take a large bowl, add oats and flour in it, stir in salt, baking powder, and coconut flakes and then whisk until combined.
4. Take another bowl, add flax seed reserve along with maple syrup, vanilla, applesauce, and milk and then whisk until combined.
5. Transfer this mixture into the oat-flour mixture, stir until combined, and fold in chocolate chips until mixed.
6. Take a skillet pan, place it over medium-low heat, spray it with oil and when hot, pour in one-fourth of the batter, spread gently into a pancake shape, and cook for 5 minutes per side until golden brown on both sides.
7. Move the pancake to your plate and repeat with the remaining batter. Serve pancakes with sliced banana.

Nutrition: *Calories: 95, Carbs: 4g, Fat: 7g, Protein: 5g*

Preparation Time: 15 minutes
Cooking Time: 15 minutes
Serving: 6

22. Chocolate Pancake

INGREDIENTS:

- 3/4 cup whole-grain flour
- 1 tablespoon ground flaxseed
- 2 tablespoons cocoa powder, unsweetened
- 1 tablespoon baking powder
- 1 tablespoon maple syrup
- 1/4 teaspoon of sea salt
- 1 tablespoon mini chocolate chips
- 1 teaspoon vanilla extract, unsweetened
- 1/4 cup applesauce, unsweetened
- 1 tablespoon apple cider vinegar
- 1 cup almond milk, unsweetened

DIRECTIONS:

1. Take a medium bowl, add flour and flaxseed in it, and then whisk in baking powder, cocoa powder, salt, and chocolate chips until well combined.
2. Take another bowl, add vanilla, maple syrup, vinegar, and milk in it, whisk until mixed and then add this mixture into the flour.
3. Add apple sauce, whisk until smooth batter comes together, and let it stand for 10 minutes at room temperature until thickened.
4. Then take a skillet pan, take a skillet pan, place it over medium heat, spray it with oil, and when hot, pour in some of the prepared batters, spread gently into a pancake shape, and cook for 3 minutes per side until golden brown on both sides.
5. Move the pancake to your plate and repeat with the remaining batter. Serve straight away.

Nutrition: *Calories: 114, Carbs: 22g, Fat: 1g, Protein: 4g*

Preparation Time: 10 minutes
Cooking Time: 30 minutes
Servings: 4

23. Vegan Corn Burger

INGREDIENTS:

- 1 tsp. green chili paste
- 1 tsp. red chili paste
- 1/4 pounds vegan cheese, grated
- Salt, to taste
- 1 tsp. vegetable oil
- 6 corns on the cob, cut in halves
- 3 oz. tomatoes, chopped
- Burger buns

DIRECTION

1. Place corn in your instant pot in a steamer basket. Add some water, cover the pot and cook on High for 10 minutes.
2. Release pressure naturally for 10 minutes.
3. Grate the cooked corn and put it in a bowl. Add cheese and stir well.
4. Set your clean instant pot on Sauté mode. Add oil and heat up.
5. Add green and red chili paste, tomatoes and salt.
6. Stir and cook for 5 minutes.
7. Spread this mix on burger buns and place them on a lined baking sheet.
8. Introduce in the oven at 350 degrees F. Bake for 5 minutes.
9. Serve with the tomato sauce you've made on top. Enjoy!

Nutrition: *calories 150, fat 28g, fiber 1g, carbs 8g, protein 8g*

Preparation Time: 10 minutes
Cooking Time: 23minutes
Servings: 4

24. Vegan Pozole

INGREDIENTS:

- 1 tbsp. olive oil
- 6 cups veggie stock
- 1 tbsp. oregano, chopped
- A pinch red pepper flakes
- 40 oz. canned jackfruit
- 14 oz. canned red chili puree
- 1 yellow onion, chopped
- 8 garlic cloves, minced
- 1 tbsp. cilantro

DIRECTION

1. Set your instant pot on Sauté mode. Add oil and heat it up.
2. Add garlic and onions. Stir and cook for 5 minutes.
3. Add chili puree, stir and cook for 1 minute more.
4. Add jackfruit, stir and cook for 2 minutes.
5. Mash this a bit and add stock.
6. Stir, cover and cook on High for 10 minutes.
7. Add oregano, cilantro and pepper flakes.
8. Stir, divide into bowls and serve. Enjoy!

Nutrition: *Calories 219 kcal Fats 13. 4g Carbs 87. 5g Protein 20 g*

Preparation Time: 6 minutes
Cooking Time: 15 minutes
Servings: 1

25. Baked Apple Breakfast Oats

INGREDIENTS:

- ⅓ cup vanilla Greek yogurt
- ⅓ cup rolled oats
- 1 apple
- 1 tbsp. peanut butter
- Touch of ground cinnamon

DIRECTIONS:

1. Preheat the air fryer oven to 350°F and press START.
2. Cut apples into chunks approximately ½-inch-thick.
3. Place apples in an oven-safe dish with some space between each chunk and sprinkle with cinnamon.
4. Select BAKE. Bake in the oven for 12 minutes
5. Combine yogurt and oats in a bowl.
6. Remove the apples from the oven and combine it with the yogurt.
7. Top with peanut butter for a delicious and high-protein breakfast.

Nutrition: *Calories 350Fat 11.2 gCarbs 52.5 gProtein 12.7 g.*

Preparation Time: 10 minutes
Cooking Time: 20 minutes
Servings: 2

26. Quinoa and Peach Bowls

INGREDIENTS:

- 2 peaches, stones removed and cubed
- 1/3 cup quinoa, rinsed
- 1 cup almond milk
- ½ teaspoon vanilla extract
- 2 teaspoons stevia

DIRECTIONS:

1. In a small pan, combine the quinoa with the peaches and the other ingredients, cover the pan and cook for 20 minutes.
2. Divide into bowls and serve

Nutrition: *calories 177, fat 2.2, fiber 4, carbs 5.4, protein 8*

Preparation Time: 10 minutes
Cooking Time: 20 minutes
Servings: 4

27. Apple Muffins

INGREDIENTS:

- ½ cup natural, unsweetened applesauce
- 1 cup apples, cored, peeled and cubed
- 2 and ½ cups old-fashioned oats
- ½ cup almond milk
- 2 tablespoons stevia
- 1 teaspoon almond extract
- Cooking spray
- 1 teaspoon cinnamon powder

DIRECTIONS:

1. In a bowl, mix the applesauce with the apples and the other ingredients except the cooking spray and stir well.
2. Divide into a muffin pan greases with cooking spray, introduce in the oven and bake at 375 degrees F for 20 minutes.
3. Serve for breakfast.

Nutrition: *calories 180, fat 4.3, fiber 4, carbs 5.4, protein 7*

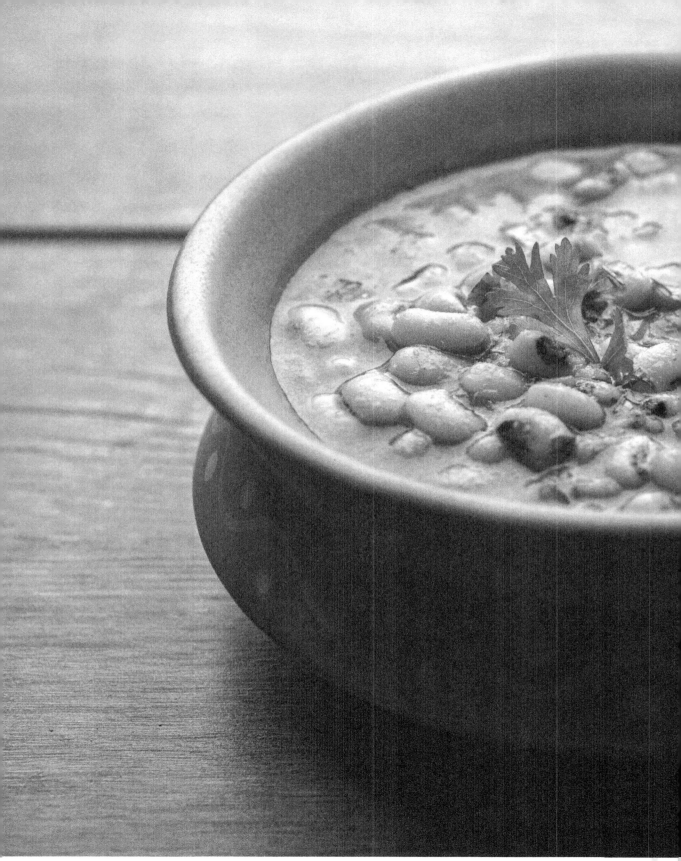

CHAPTER 4:
MAIN DISHES

Preparation Time: 10 minutes
Cooking Time: 13 minutes
Serving: 2

28. Spiced Okra

INGREDIENTS:

- 1 tablespoon avocado oil
- ¾ pound okra pods, 2-inch pieces
- ½ teaspoon ground cumin
- ½ teaspoon cayenne powder
- Sea salt, as required

DIRECTIONS:

1. Cook the oil over medium heat and stir fry the okra for about 2 minutes. Reduce the heat to low and cook covered for about 6-8 minutes stirring occasionally.
2. Add the cumin, cayenne powder and salt and stir to combine. Increase the heat to medium and cook uncovered for about 2-3 minutes more. Remove from the heat and serve hot.

Nutrition: *calories 280, fat 8, fiber 3, carbs 8, protein 6*

Preparation Time: 15 minutes
Cooking Time: 15 minutes
Servings: 4

29. Bell Peppers & Zucchini Stir Fry

INGREDIENTS:

- 2 tablespoons avocado oil
- 1 large onion, cubed
- 4 garlic cloves, minced
- 1 large green bell pepper
- 1 large red bell pepper
- 1 large yellow bell pepper
- 2 cups zucchini, sliced
- ¼ cup spring water
- Sea salt, as required
- Cayenne powder, as required

DIRECTIONS:

1. Cook the oil over medium heat and sauté the onion and garlic for about 4-5 minutes. Add the vegetables and stir fry for about 4-5 minutes. Add the water and stir fry for about 3-4 minutes more. Serve hot.

Nutrition: *calories 207, fat 8, fiber 2, carbs 8, protein 6*

30. Spanish rice

Preparation Time: 10 minutes
Cooking Time: 40 minutes
Servings: 10

INGREDIENTS:

- 1 cup of long grain rice, uncooked
- 1/2 cup of chopped green bell pepper
- 14 ounce of diced tomatoes
- 1/2 cup of chopped white onion
- 1 teaspoon of minced garlic
- 1/2 teaspoon of salt
- 1 teaspoon of red chili powder
- 1 teaspoon of ground cumin
- 4-ounce of tomato puree
- 8 fluid ounce of water

DIRECTIONS:

1. Grease a 6-quarts slow cooker with a non-stick cooking spray and add all the ingredients into it.
2. Stir properly and cover the top.
3. Plug in the slow cooker; adjust the cooking time to 5 hours and let it cook on the high heat setting or until the rice absorbs all the liquid.
4. Serve right away.

Nutrition: *calories 340, fat 8, fiber 2, carbs 8, protein 6*

31. Super tasty Vegetarian Chili

Preparation Time: 10 minutes
Cooking Time: 45 minutes
Servings: 6

INGREDIENTS:

- 16-ounce of vegetarian baked beans
- 16 ounce of cooked chickpeas
- 16 ounce of cooked kidney beans
- 15 ounce of cooked corn
- 1 medium-sized green bell pepper, cored and chopped
- 2 stalks of celery, peeled and chopped
- 12 ounce of chopped tomatoes
- 1 medium-sized white onion, peeled and chopped
- 1 teaspoon of minced garlic
- 1 teaspoon of salt
- 1 tablespoon of red chili powder
- 1 tablespoon of dried oregano
- 1 tablespoon of dried basil
- 1 tablespoon of dried parsley
- 18-ounce of black bean soup
- 4-ounce of tomato puree

DIRECTIONS:

1. Take a 6-quarts slow cooker, grease it with a non-stick cooking spray and place all the ingredients into it.
2. Stir properly and cover the top.
3. Plug in the slow cooker; adjust the cooking time to 2 hours and let it cook on the high heat setting or until it is cooked thoroughly.
4. Serve right away.

Nutrition: *calories 340, fat 8, fiber 2, carbs 8, protein 6*

Preparation Time: 30 minutes
Cooking Time: 15 minutes
Servings: 6

32. Quinoa and Black Bean Lettuce Wraps

INGREDIENTS:

- 2 tablespoons avocado oil (optional)
- ¼ cup deseeded and chopped bell pepper
- ½ onion, chopped
- 2 tablespoons minced garlic
- 1 teaspoon salt (optional)
- 1 teaspoon pepper (optional)
- ½ cup cooked quinoa
- 1 cup cooked black beans
- ½ cup almond flour
- ½ teaspoon paprika
- ½ teaspoon red pepper flakes
- 6 large lettuce leaves

Nutrition: *calories: 200 fat: 10.6g carbs: 40.5g protein: 9.5g fiber: 8.2g*

DIRECTIONS:

1. Heat 1 tablespoon of the avocado oil (if desired) in a skillet over medium-high heat.
2. Add the bell peppers, onions, garlic, salt (if desired), and pepper. Sauté for 5 minutes or until the bell peppers are tender.
3. Turn off the heat and allow to cool for 10 minutes, then pour the vegetables in a food processor. Add the quinoa, beans, flour. Sprinkle with paprika and red pepper flakes. Pulse until thick and well combined.
4. Line a baking pan with parchment paper, then shape the mixture into 6 patties with your hands and place on the baking pan.
5. Put the fpan in the freezer for 5 minutes to make the patties firm.
6. Heat the remaining avocado oil (if desired) in the skillet over high heat.
7. Add the patties and cook for 6 minutes or until well browned on both sides. Flip the patties halfway through.
8. Arrange the patties in the lettuce leaves and serve immediately.

33. Rice and Bean Lettuce Burgers

Preparation Time: 15 minutes
Cooking Time: 45 minutes
Servings: 8

INGREDIENTS:

- 1 cup uncooked medium-grain brown rice
- 2 cups water
- ½ cup grated carrots
- ¾ cup chopped red onion
- ½ cup raw sunflower seeds
- ¾ cup cooked pinto beans
- 5 cloves garlic, peeled
- 2 tablespoons oat flour
- 2 teaspoons arrowroot powder
- 2 tablespoons nutritional yeast
- ¼ cup chopped fresh basil
- 4 teaspoons ground cumin
- 4 teaspoons low-sodium soy sauce
- 2 tablespoons low -sodium tomato paste
- Salt and ground black pepper, to taste (optional)
- 1 to 2 tablespoons water
- 8 large lettuce leaves, for serving

Nutrition: *calories: 197 fat: 5.9g carbs: 30.5g protein: 7.4g fiber: 4.7g*

DIRECTION:

1. Pour the rice and water in a pot. Bring to a boil over medium heat. Reduce the heat to low and simmer for 15 more minutes or until the rice is tender. Transfer the rice in a large bowl. Allow the rice to cool and fluff with a fork.
2. Put the carrots, onions, sunflower seeds, beans, and garlic in a food processor and pulse until well combined and chunky. Pour the mixture over the rice.
3. Add the remaining ingredients, except for the lettuce, to the bowl of rice, then toss to combine well. Shape the mixture into 8 patties and arrange them on a parchment-lined baking pan. Refrigerate for an hour until firm.
4. Preheat the oven to 350°F (180°C).
5. Place the baking pan in the oven and bake for 30 minutes or until well browned on both sides. Flip the patties halfway through.
6. Unfold the lettuce leaves on 8 plates, then top each leaf with a patty. Wrap and serve.

Preparation Time: 10 minutes
Cooking Time: 25 minutes
Servings: 4

34. Mexican Portobello Mushrooms

INGREDIENTS:

- 4 large portobello mushrooms (without stems)
- 1 cup of black beans (drained)
- 1 cup of guacamole
- ¼ cup black olives
- ¼ cup of Rosa tomatoes (chopped)
- Nacho cheese:
- ½ cup of cashews (softened)
- 1 cup of water
- 3 tbsp of nutritional yeast
- 3 tbsp of tapioca starch
- 2 tbsp of lemon juice
- 1 ½ tsp of salt
- 1 tsp of agave nectar
- 1 tsp of paprika
- ½ tsp of garlic powder
- ¼ cup of turmeric

Nutrition: *Calories: 218, Carbohydrates: 22g, Protein: 7g, Fat: 12g*

DIRECTIONS:

1. Soften the cashews by boiling them on high heat for 10 minutes, drain it, and then blending it with the remaining ingredients until it reaches the desired consistency.
2. Once done, strain it until there are no cashew bits left in the sauce, and then cook it in a saucepan over medium heat while stirring it continuously for 5 minutes.
3. Add the black beans and tomatoes to the cheese sauce on the stove, and mix well. Prep a baking sheet by adding a parchment paper layer to it, and place the portobello mushrooms onto the sheet.
4. Divide the cheese sauce bean mixture evenly between the 4 mushrooms, and fill it until full. Bake the mushrooms at 375 degrees-Fahrenheit for 15 minutes.
5. Once it is finished cooking, serve the mushrooms with black olives and a heaping tbsp of guacamole. Alternatively, store the mushrooms in an airtight container, and refrigerate them for 2 days.

Preparation Time: 20 minutes
Cooking Time: 20 minutes
Servings: 4

35. Potato Tempeh Hash

INGREDIENTS:

- 4 medium potatoes
- 1 8 oz package of tempeh (diced)
- 6 kale leaves (steamed and chopped)
- 1 green bell pepper (diced)
- 1 onion (diced)
- 2 tbsp of nutritional yeast
- 2 tbsp of olive oil
- 1 tsp of cilantro
- 1 tsp of black pepper
- Sriracha (optional)

Nutrition: *Calories: 269, Carbohydrates: 44g, Protein: 9g, Fat: 8g*

DIRECTIONS:

1. Bake the potatoes in the microwave for 5-6 minutes or until cooked yet firm. Once cooled down, pull the skin off and dispose of it. Then, chop the potato into small cubes.
2. Add olive oil to a large pan, and cook the onion over medium heat for 1 to 2 minutes. Then, add the steamed kale, cubed potato, cilantro, and black pepper to the pan, and mix everything.
3. Put the nutritional yeast, then continue stirring until everything is well combined. Serve hot with sriracha sauce, divide the potato tempeh hash between 4 containers, and refrigerate it for up to 3 days.

Preparation Time: 10 minutes
Cooking Time: 20 minutes
Servings: 4

36. Vegan Spinach Pasta

INGREDIENTS

- 2 garlic cloves, chopped
- A drizzle olive oil
- Salt and black pepper, to taste
- 1/4 cup pine nuts, chopped
- 1 pound spinach
- 1 pound fusilli pasta
- 2 garlic cloves, crushed
- Vegan cheese, grated for serving

DIRECTION

1. Set the instant pot on Sauté mode. Add olive oil and heat up.
2. Add spinach and crushed garlic. Stir and cook for 6 to 8 minutes.
3. Add pasta, salt and pepper to taste. Add some water to cover the pasta.
4. Stir and cook on Low for 6 minutes.
5. Release pressure, add chopped garlic and pine nuts.
6. Stir, divide amongst plates and serve with grated vegan cheese on top. Enjoy!

Nutrition: *Calories: 379; Total fat: 5g; Carbs: 6g; Fiber: 2g; Protein: 4g*

Preparation Time: 10 minutes
Cooking Time: 6 minutes
Servings: 4

37. White Couscous with Syrup

INGREDIENTS:

- 1/3 cup maple syrup
- 1/3 teaspoon ground cinnamon
- 1 cup white couscous
- 1 teaspoon almond butter
- 2 cups of water

DIRECTIONS:

1. Pour water in the instant pot.
2. Add almond butter and couscous.
3. Close the lid and cook on Manual mode (High pressure) for 6 minutes.
4. Then make quick pressure release and transfer cooked couscous in the bowl.
5. Add maple syrup and ground cinnamon and stir well.

Nutrition: *calories 252, fat 2.6, fiber 2.7, carbs 52, protein 6.4*

Preparation Time: 10 minutes
Cooking Time: 25 minutes
Servings: 4

38. Sautéed Collard Greens

INGREDIENTS:

- 1½ pounds collard greens
- 1 cup vegetable broth
- ½ teaspoon garlic powder
- ½ teaspoon onion powder
- ⅛ teaspoon freshly ground black pepper

DIRECTIONS:

1. Remove the hard middle stems from the greens, then roughly chop the leaves into 2-inch pieces.
2. In a large saucepan, mix together the vegetable broth, garlic powder, onion powder, and pepper. Bring to a boil over medium-high heat, then add the chopped greens. Reduce the heat to low, and cover.
3. Cook for 20 minutes, stirring well every 4 to 5 minutes, and serve. (If you notice that the liquid has completely evaporated and the greens are beginning to stick to the bottom of the pan, stir in a few extra tablespoons of vegetable broth or water.)

Nutrition: *Calories: 28; Total fat: 1g; Carbohydrates: 4g; Fiber: 2g; Protein: 3g*

Preparation Time: 15 minutes
Cooking Time: 0 minutes
Servings: 4

39. Creamy Chickpea Sandwiches

INGREDIENTS:

- 8 slices of rye bread
- 4 romaine lettuce leaves
- 2 medium stalks of celery (chopped)
- 1 can of chickpeas (drained)
- ¼ cup of onion (diced)
- ½ tsp of black pepper
- Sandwich dressing:
- ¼ cup of vegan mayo
- 1 tsp of apple cider vinegar
- ½ tsp of basil
- ½ tsp of chives
- ½ tsp of Himalayan salt
- ¼ tsp of onion powder

DIRECTIONS:

1. Mix the sandwich dressing ingredients in a bowl. Add the chickpeas to the dressing, and mash it using a fork. Add the celery, onion, and black pepper to the chickpea-dressing mixture, and remix everything.
2. Toast the rye bread, and spread 4 slices thereof with the chickpea-dressing mixture. Cover it with another slice of rye bread, and serve it immediately or store it in Ziploc bags for up to 2 days.

Nutrition: *Calories: 380, Carbohydrates: 54g, Protein: 18g, Fat: 27g*

Preparation Time: 15 Minutes
Cooking Time: 8 hours
Servings: 8

40. Flavorful Refried Beans

INGREDIENTS:

- 3 cups of pinto beans, rinsed
- 1 small jalapeno pepper, seeded and chopped
- 1 medium-sized white onion, peeled and sliced
- 2 tablespoons of minced garlic
- 5 teaspoons of salt
- 2 teaspoons of ground black pepper
- 1/4 teaspoon of ground cumin
- 9 cups of water

DIRECTIONS:

1. Using a 6-quarts slow cooker, place all the Ingredients: and stir until it mixes properly.
2. Cover the top, plug in the slow cooker; adjust the cooking time to 6 hours, let it cook on high heat setting and add more water if the beans get too dry.
3. When the beans are done, drain them and reserve the liquid.
4. Mash the beans using a potato masher and pour in the reserved cooking liquid until it reaches your desired mixture.
5. Serve immediately.

Nutrition: *Calories: 198; Carbs: 22g; Fat: 7g; Protein: 19g*

Preparation Time: 15 Minutes
Cooking Time: 5 hours
Servings: 8

41. Smoky Red Beans and Rice

INGREDIENTS:

- 30 ounce of cooked red beans
- 1 cup of brown rice, uncooked
- 1 cup of chopped green pepper
- 1 cup of chopped celery
- 1 cup of chopped white onion
- 1 1/2 teaspoon of minced garlic
- 1/2 teaspoon of salt
- 1/4 teaspoon of cayenne pepper
- 1 teaspoon of smoked paprika
- 2 teaspoons of dried thyme
- 1 bay leaf
- 2 1/3 cups of vegetable broth

DIRECTIONS:

1. Using a 6-quarts slow cooker place all the Ingredients: except for the rice, salt and cayenne pepper.
2. Stir until it mixes properly and then cover the top.
3. Plug in the slow cooker; adjust the cooking time to 4 hours and let it steam on a low heat setting.
4. Then pour in and stir the rice, salt, cayenne pepper and continue cooking for an additional 2 hours at a high heat setting.

Nutrition: *Calories: 234; Carbs: 13g; Fat: 7g; Protein: 19g*

Preparation Time: 15 Minutes
Cooking Time: 60 Minutes
Servings: 8

42. Spicy Black-Eyed Peas

INGREDIENTS:

- 32-ounce black-eyed peas, un-cooked
- 1 cup of chopped orange bell pepper
- 1 cup of chopped celery
- 8-ounce of chipotle peppers, chopped
- 1 cup of chopped carrot
- 1 cup of chopped white onion
- 1 teaspoon of minced garlic
- 3/4 teaspoon of salt
- 1/2 teaspoon of ground black pepper
- 2 teaspoons of liquid smoke flavoring
- 2 teaspoons of ground cumin
- 1 tablespoon of adobo sauce
- 2 tablespoons of olive oil
- 1 tablespoon of apple cider vinegar
- 4 cups of vegetable broth

DIRECTIONS:

1. Place a medium-sized non-stick skillet pan over an average temperature of heat; add the bell peppers, carrot, onion, garlic, oil and vinegar.
2. Stir until it mixes properly and let it cook for 5 to 8 minutes or until it gets translucent.
3. Transfer this mixture to a 6-quarts slow cooker and add the peas, chipotle pepper, adobo sauce and the vegetable broth.
4. Stir until mixes properly and cover the top.
5. Plug in the slow cooker; adjust the cooking time to 8 hours and let it cook on the low heat setting or until peas are soft.

Nutrition: *Calories: 211; Carbs: 22g; Fat: 7g; Protein: 19g*

Preparation Time: 10 minutes
Cooking Time: 30 minutes
Servings: 4

43. Coconut Mushroom Pizza

INGREDIENTS:

- 1 ½ cups of coconut milk
- 1 ¾ cup of button mushrooms (sliced)
- 2 cloves of garlic (minced)
- 1 pack of pre-made pizza dough (gluten-free)
- ½ onion (diced)
- 1 tbsp of vegan butter
- 1 tbsp of flour (all-purpose)
- 1 tbsp of olive oil
- 1 tsp of black pepper
- 1 tsp of thyme
- 1 tsp of salt

DIRECTIONS:

1. Heat the oven to 425 degrees-Fahrenheit, and spray a pizza pan with non-stick cooking spray. Add 1 tbsp olive oil to a medium-large pan, and cook the garlic and onion over high heat for 2 minutes.
2. Add the mushrooms to the pan, and cook them for 5 minutes. Stir the mushrooms frequently to prevent them from sticking to the pan.
3. Once done, remove the ingredients from the pan and set it aside to cool down. Add 1 tbsp of vegan butter to the pan, and stir in the flour. Mix the ingredients for 1 minute to form a paste.
4. Add the coconut milk, and whisk the pan ingredients for 5 minutes. Once the sauce is thick, remove it from the heat.
5. Prepare the pizza by stretching the store-bought dough out on a flat surface and dusting it on both sides with added flour.
6. Once done, place the mushrooms on top of the pizza dough, and drizzle the sauce over the entire pizza.
7. Bake the pizza in the oven within 20 minutes and cool down for 10 minutes before slicing it. Serve hot. Alternatively, store it in a container for 2 to 3 days.

Nutrition: *Calories: 460, Carbohydrates: 56g, Protein: 12g, Fat: 18g*

Preparation Time: 5 minutes
Cooking Time: 25 minutes
Servings: 4

44. Sweet Potato Chickpea Wraps

INGREDIENTS:

- 4 flatbreads (gluten-free)
- 15 oz of chickpeas (drained and rinsed)
- 2 large sweet potatoes (washed, peeled, & cubed)
- 1 cup of arugula
- 4 tbsp of plain hummus
- 2 tbsp of avocado oil
- 2 tbsp of pumpkin seeds
- 2 tbsp of dried cranberries
- 2 tsp of thyme
- 1 tsp of cilantro
- 1 tsp of sea salt
- ¼ tsp of red chili powder
- ¼ tsp of cinnamon

Nutrition: *Calories: 460, Carbohydrates: 80g, Protein: 12g, Fat: 9.8g*

DIRECTIONS:

1. Set the oven to 400 degrees-Fahrenheit. Add avocado oil, cinnamon, sea salt, thyme, cilantro, and red chili powder to a mixing bowl, and combine them.
2. Add the sweet potatoes and chickpeas to the mixing bowl, and mix them with the seasoning until everything is covered.
3. Spread the marinated sweet potato and chickpeas onto the baking sheet, and bake it for 25 minutes. Flip the ingredients 15 min in.
4. Turn it over to cook on the other side for the remaining 10 minutes. Remove the baking sheet from the oven. Assemble the flatbreads by spreading each with a medium layer of hummus.
5. Divide the sweet potatoes and chickpeas between 4 flatbreads and place them in the center, followed by arugula, pumpkin seeds, and cranberries.
6. Close the flatbread by rolling it up into a wrap. Refrigerate the wraps in a container for 3 days.

Preparation Time: 15 minutes
Cooking Time: 25 minutes
Servings: 4

45. Vegan Burgers

INGREDIENTS:

- 4 slider buns (gluten-free)
- 2 garlic cloves (minced)
- 1 ¼ cup of pinto beans
- 1 ¼ cup of black beans
- 1 cup of corn
- 1 green bell pepper (diced)
- ½ green onion
- ¼ cup of water
- ¼ cup of peppadews (seeded and diced)
- 4 tbsp of guacamole
- 2 tbsp of parsley
- 1 tbsp of olive oil
- Burger sauce: 12 oz of salsa, ¼ cup of brown sugar, 1 tbsp of red chili flakes, 2 tsp of paprika, 1 tsp of thyme, and ½ tsp of black pepper

DIRECTIONS:

1. Mix the burger sauce fixings in a bowl, and set it aside. Put the diced onion in your large pan with olive oil, and allow it to cook for 3 minutes. Once done, add the minced garlic, and let it cook for 1 minute.
2. Add the green bell pepper and peppadews to the pan, and cook for 4 minutes. Then, add the water to the pan. Add the mixed burger sauce to the pan. Simmer for 10 minutes.
3. Put the corn, black beans, plus pinto beans. Combine all the ingredients in the pan—Cook for 5 more minutes. Add the parsley to the bean-corn mixture and cook for 1 minute.
4. Plate the slider buns, and add the mixture to the buns, distributing it evenly. Serve with 1 tbsp of guacamole each.

Nutrition: *Calories: 220, Carbohydrates: 39g, Protein: 9g, Fat: 2.5g*

Preparation Time: 5 minutes
Cooking Time: 10 minutes
Servings: 4

46. Black Bean Kale Salad Jars

INGREDIENTS:

- 6 cups of kale (prepped and shredded)
- 19 oz of black beans (drained)
- 2 garlic cloves (minced)
- 1 red bell pepper (diced)
- ½ red onion (diced)
- 4 tbsp of red pepper hummus
- 2 tbsp of tomato paste
- 1 tsp of cilantro
- 1 tsp of agave
- ½ tsp of black pepper

DIRECTIONS:

1. Put olive oil into your large non-stick pan. Next, add the beans over medium-high heat, and cook them for 5 minutes before adding the diced onions and garlic. Cook for 4 to 5 minutes.
2. Add the bell pepper, tomato paste, cilantro, agave, and black pepper to the pan, combine the ingredients, and allow it to simmer for 4 minutes.
3. Assemble the ingredients in 4 mason jars by placing shredded kale in each jar, filling it a ¼ full.
4. Add the bean mixture to the jars until the jar is half full. Add ½ tbsp of hummus on top, and repeat the three steps until the jars are full.
5. Add extra black pepper and salt if needed; close the airtight jars. Put them in the refrigerator for 3 days. Serve cold.

Nutrition: *Calories: 290, Carbohydrates: 33g, Protein: 11g, Fat: 7.7g*

Preparation Time: 30 minutes
Cooking Time: 10 minutes
Servings: 8

47. Bulgur and Pinto Bean Lettuce Wraps

INGREDIENTS:

- 1½ cups plus 2 tablespoons water, divided
- Salt and ground black pepper, to taste (optional)
- ⅔ cup bulgur, rinsed
- ¾ cup walnuts
- ½ cup fresh basil leaves
- 2 garlic cloves, minced
- 1 large beet (about 9 ounces / 255 g), peeled and shredded
- 1 (15-ounce / 425-g) can pinto beans, rinsed
- 1 (4-ounce / 113-g) jar carrot
- 1 tablespoon Dijon mustard
- 1½ cups panko bread crumbs
- 6 tablespoons avocado oil (optional)
- 8 large lettuce leaves

DIRECTION:

1. Pour 1½ cups of water in a pot and sprinkle with salt (if desired) to taste. Bring to a boil, then turn off the heat. Pour the bulgur in the boiling water. Cover the lid and let sit for 15 minutes or until the bulgur is soft. Drain the bulgur and spread it on a baking pan to cool.
2. Meanwhile, combine the walnuts, basil, garlic, and beet in a food processor. Pulse to mix well. Then add the beans, carrot, 2 tablespoons of water, Dijon mustard, salt (if desired) and pepper. Pulse to combine well.
3. Pour the mixture in a large bowl and fold in the cooked bulgur and panko. Shape the mixture into 8 patties.
4. Heat the avocado oil (if desired) in the skillet over medium-high heat.
5. Arrange the patties in a skillet and cook for 8 minutes or until well browned on both sides. Flip the patties halfway through. Work in batches to avoid overcrowding.
6. Unfold the lettuce leaves on 8 plates, then top the leaves with the patties and wrap to serve.

Nutrition: *calories: 317 fat: 17.2g carbs: 33.9gprotein: 8.9gfiber: 6.5g*

Preparation Time: 20 minutes
Cooking Time: 4 hours
Servings: 4

48. Barbecued Greens & Grits

INGREDIENTS:

- 14 oz. tempeh, sliced
- 3 c. vegetable broth
- 3 c. collard greens, chopped
- ½ c. BBQ sauce
- 1 c. gluten-free grits
- ¼ c. white onion, diced
- 2 tbsps. olive oil
- 2 garlic cloves, minced
- 1 tsp. salt

DIRECTIONS:

1 Preheat the oven to 400°F.

2. Mix tempeh slices with the BBQ sauce in a shallow baking dish. Set aside and let marinate for up to 3 hours.

3. Heat 1 tablespoon of olive oil in a frying pan over medium heat, then add the garlic and sauté until fragrant.

4. Add the collard greens and ½ teaspoon of salt and cook until the collards are wilted and dark. Set the pan from heat and set aside.

5. Cover the tempeh and BBQ sauce mixture with aluminum foil. In your oven, set the baking dish in place and bake the ingredients for 15 minutes. Uncover and continue to bake for another 10 minutes until the tempeh is browned and crispy.

6. While the tempeh cooks heat the remaining tablespoon of olive oil in the previously used frying pan over medium heat.

7. Cook the onions until brown and fragrant, around 10 minutes.

8. Pour in the vegetable broth and bring it to a boil; then turn the heat down to low.

9. Slowly whisk the grits into the simmering broth. Add the remaining ½ teaspoon of salt before covering the pan with a lid.

10. Let the ingredients simmer for about 8 minutes until the grits are soft and creamy.

11. Serve the tempeh and collard greens on top of a bowl of grits and enjoy, or store for later!

Nutrition: *Calories 374, Fat 19.1g, Carbs 31.1g, Protein 23.7g*

Preparation Time: 10 minutes
Cooking Time: 30 minutes
Servings: 12

49. Chickpea and Spinach Cutlets

INGREDIENTS:

- 1 Red Bell Pepper
- 19 oz. Chickpeas, Rinsed & Drained
- 1 c. ground Almonds
- 2 tsps. Dijon Mustard
- 1 tsp. Oregano
- ½ tsp. Sage
- 1 c. Spinach, Fresh
- 1½ c. Rolled Oats
- 1 Clove Garlic, Pressed
- ½ Lemon, Juiced
- 2 tsps. Maple Syrup, Pure

Nutrition: *Calories: 200, Protein: 8 g, Fat: 11g, Carbs: 21 g*

DIRECTIONS:

1. Get out a baking sheet. Line it with parchment paper.
2. Cut your red pepper in half and then take the seeds out. Place it on your baking sheet, and roast in the oven while you prepare your other ingredients.
3. Process your chickpeas, almonds, mustard, and maple syrup together in a food processor.
4. Add in your lemon juice, oregano, sage, garlic, and spinach, processing again. Make sure it's combined, but don't puree it.
5. Once your red bell pepper is softened, which should roughly take ten minutes, add this to the processor as well. Add in your oats, mixing well.
6. Form twelve patties, cooking in the oven for a half hour. They should be browned.

Preparation Time: 10 minutes
Cooking Time: 0 minutes
Servings: 4

50. Chickpea and Mayonnaise Salad Sandwich

INGREDIENTS:

- For the mayonnaise:
- 1/3 cup cashew nuts, soaked in boiling water for 10 minutes
- ½ teaspoon ground black pepper
- 1 teaspoon salt
- 6 teaspoons apple cider vinegar
- 2 teaspoon maple syrup
- 1/2 teaspoon Dijon mustard
- For the chickpea salad:
- 1 small bunch of chives, chopped
- 1 ½ cup sweetcorn
- 3 cups cooked chickpeas
- To serve:
- 4 sandwich bread
- 4 leaves of lettuce
- ½ cup chopped cherry tomatoes

DIRECTIONS:

1. Prepare the mayonnaise and for this, place all of its ingredients in a food processor and then pulse for 2 minutes until smooth, scraping the sides of the container frequently.
2. Take a medium bowl, place chickpeas in it, and then mash by using a fork until broken.
3. Add chives and corn, stir until mixed, then add mayonnaise and stir until well combined.
4. Assemble the sandwich and for this, stuff sandwich bread with chickpea salad, top each sandwich with a lettuce leaf, and ¼ cup of chopped tomatoes and then serve.

Nutrition: *calories 163, fat 8g, fiber 2g, carbs 8g, protein 11g*

Preparation Time: 10 minutes
Cooking Time: 12 minutes
Servings: 4

51. Coconut Mushroom Dumplings

INGREDIENTS:

- 1 lb. ground mushroom
- 2 scallions, chopped
- 1 small cucumber, deseeded and grated
- 4 garlic cloves, minced
- 1 tsp freshly pureed ginger
- 1 tsp red chili flakes
- 2 tbsp tamari sauce
- 2 tbsp sesame oil
- 3 tbsp coconut oil, for frying

DIRECTIONS:

1. In a medium bowl, combine the mushroom, scallions, cucumber, garlic, ginger, red chili flakes, tamari sauce, and sesame oil. Using your hands, form 1-inch oval shapes out of the mixture and place them on a plate.
2. Heat the coconut oil in a medium skillet over medium heat; fry the dumplings for 12 minutes until brown on both sides and cooked
3. Transfer to a paper towel-lined plate to drain grease and serve with creamy spinach puree.

Nutrition: *Calories: 439; Total Fat: 31.9g; Saturated Fat: 12.2g; Total Carbs: 9g; Dietary Fiber: 4g; Sugar: 1g; Protein: 36g; Sodium: 574mg*

Preparation Time: 10 minutes
Cooking Time: 5 minutes
Servings: 4

52. Mushrooms Sandwich

INGREDIENTS:

- 8 cherry tomatoes, halved
- 2 ounces of baby spinach
- 20 ounces of oyster mushrooms
- 2/3 teaspoon salt
- 1/3 teaspoon ground black pepper
- 2 tablespoons olive oil
- 4 tablespoons of barbecue sauce
- 8 slices of bread, toasted

DIRECTIONS:

1. Take a griddle pan, place it over medium-high heat, grease it with oil and let it preheat.
2. Cut mushroom into thin strips, add to the hot griddle pan, drizzle with oil and cook for 5 minutes until done.
3. Transfer grilled mushrooms into a medium bowl, season with salt and black pepper, add barbecue sauce and toss until mixed.
4. Spread prepared mushroom mixture evenly on four bread slices, top with spinach and cherry tomatoes, then cover with the other four slices and serve.

Nutrition: *calories 200, fat 8g, fiber 2g, carbs 8g, protein 6g*

Preparation Time: 10 minutes
Cooking Time: 0 minutes
Serving: 4

53. Rainbow Taco Boats

INGREDIENTS:

- 1 head romaine lettuce,
- For the Filling:
- 1/2 cup alfalfa sprouts
- 1 medium avocado, peeled, pitted, cubed
- 1 cup shredded carrots
- 1 cup halved cherry tomatoes
- 3/4 cup sliced red cabbage
- 1/2 cup sprouted hummus dip
- 1 tablespoon hemp seeds
- For the Sauce:
- 1 tablespoon maple syrup
- 1/3 cup tahini
- 1/8 teaspoon sea salt
- 2 tablespoons lemon juice
- 3 tablespoons water

DIRECTIONS:

1. Prepare the sauce and for this, take a medium bowl, add all the ingredients in it and whisk until well combined.
2. Assemble the boats and for this, arrange lettuce leaves in twelve portions, top each with hummus, and the remaining ingredients for the filling.
3. Serve with prepared sauce.

Nutrition: *calories 443, fat 8g, fiber1g, carbs 8g, protein 3g*

Preparation Time: 10 minutes
Cooking Time: 8 hours
Servings: 8

54. Scrumptious Baked Potatoes

INGREDIENTS:

- 8 potatoes
- Salt to taste for serving
- Ground black pepper to taste for serving

DIRECTIONS:

1. Rinse potatoes until clean, wipe dry and then prick with a fork.
2. Wrap each potato in an aluminum foil and place in a 6 to 8 quarts slow cooker.
3. Cover with lid, and then plug in the slow cooker and let cook on low heat setting for 8 hours or until tender.
4. When the cooking time is over, unwrap potatoes and prick with a fork to check if potatoes are tender or not.
5. Sprinkle potatoes with salt, black pepper, and your favorite seasoning and serve.

Nutrition: *calories 350, fat 28g, fiber 1g, carbs 8g, protein 22g*

Preparation Time: 15 minutes
Cooking Time: 4 hours
Servings: 6

55. Fantastic Butternut Squash & Vegetables

INGREDIENTS:

- 1-1/2 cups of corn kernels
- 2 pounds of butternut squash
- 1 medium-sized green bell pepper
- 14-1/2 ounce of diced tomatoes
- 1/2 cup of chopped white onion
- 1/2 teaspoon of minced garlic
- 1/2 teaspoon of salt
- 1/4 teaspoon of ground black pepper
- 1 tablespoon and 2 teaspoons of tomato paste
- 1/2 cup of vegetable broth

DIRECTIONS:

1. Peel, centralize the butternut squash and dice, and place it into a 6-quarts slow cooker. Create a hole on the green bell pepper, then cut it into 1/2-inch pieces and add it to the slow cooker. Add the remaining ingredients into the slow cooker except for tomato paste, stir properly and cover it with the lid.
2. Turn on the slow cooker and cook on low heat setting for 6 hours. When 6 hours of the cooking time is done, remove 1/2 cup of the cooking liquid from the slow cooker. Then pour the tomatoes mixture into this cooking liquid, stir properly and place it in the slow cooker.
3. Stir properly and continue cooking for 30 minutes or until the mixture becomes slightly thick. Serve right away.

Nutrition: *calories 350, fat 28g, fiber 1g, carbs 8g, protein 22g*

Preparation Time: 10 minutes
Cooking Time: 30 minutes
Servings: 4

56. Couscous with Mint

INGREDIENTS:

- 1 cup pearl couscous
- 2 tbsps. extra virgin olive oil
- 1 small yellow onion, thinly sliced
- 1 and ½ cups veggie stock
- 2/3 cup green peas
- ¼ cup cheese, grated
- 2 tbsps. mint leaves, finely chopped
- Salt and black pepper to the taste

DIRECTIONS:

1. Heat oil on Sauté. Add onion and cook for 3 minutes. Add stock, couscous, peas, salt, and pepper. Stir and cover. Cook on High for 5 minutes. Open and add cheese and mint. Mix and serve.

Nutrition: *calories 357, fat 14.8, fiber 2.8, carbs 51.7, protein 5.8*

57. Cowboy Caviar

Servings: 4

INGREDIENTS:

- ½ black-eyed peas
- 1 cup of water
- 4 tomatoes, chopped
- 1 tablespoon apple cider vinegar
- 1 tablespoon lemon juice
- 1 jalapeno pepper, chopped
- ½ cup fresh parsley, chopped
- 2 tablespoons olive oil
- ½ teaspoon salt

DIRECTIONS:

1. In the instant pot combine together black-eyed peas and water. Close the lid.
2. Set manual mode and cook on Pressure for 6 minutes. Then make quick pressure release.
3. In the mixing bowl mix up together chopped tomatoes, jalapeno pepper, parsley, and apple cider vinegar.
4. When the black-eyed peas are chilled, add them in the tomato mixture.
5. Add olive oil, salt, and lemon juice.
6. Mix up the caviar carefully before serving.

Nutrition: *calories 99, fat 7.5, fiber 2.4, carbs 7.6, protein 2.1*

58. Creamy Mushroom Alfredo Rice

INGREDIENTS:

- 1 cup of rice
- 2 tbsps. olive oil
- 2 ¾ cups of vegetable stock
- ¾ cup onions, finely chopped
- 2 garlic cloves, minced
- 1½ tbsps. fresh lemon juice
- 2 oz. creamy mushroom Alfredo sauce
- Salt and black pepper, to taste
- ¼ cup walnuts, coarsely chopped

DIRECTIONS:

1. Put the oil, onions, and garlic in the pot and press Sauté. Sauté for 3 minutes and add rice and broth. Cover and cook on High for 22 minutes. Open and add lemon juice, salt, pepper, and sauce. Garnish and serve

Nutrition: *calories 304, fat 10.3, fiber 5.4, carbs 46.8, protein 8.4*

Preparation Time: 10 minutes
Cooking Time: 30 minutes
Servings: 4

59. Curried Sorghum

INGREDIENTS:

- 3 cups of water
- 1 cup sorghum
- 1 cup milk
- Salt to the taste
- 3 tbsps. rice wine vinegar
- ½ tsp. chili powder
- 1 tbsp. curry powder
- 2 cups carrots
- ½ cup golden raisins
- ¼ cup green onion, finely chopped
- 2 tsps. sugar

DIRECTIONS:

1. Put the sorghum, water, and salt in the pot. Cover and cook on High for 20 minutes. In a bowl, mix sugar, milk, vinegar, salt, curry powder, and chili powder and mix well.
2. Drain sorghum and transfer to a bowl.
3. Add milk mix, carrots, onions, and raisins. Mix and serve.

Nutrition: *calories 304, fat 10.3, fiber 5.4, carbs 46.8, protein 8.4*

Preparation Time: 10 minutes
Cooking Time: 30 minutes
Servings: 4

60. Kidney beans with Veggies

INGREDIENTS:

- 1 cup kidney beans, soaked overnight
- 1 medium carrot, chopped
- 1 cup tomatoes, chopped
- 3 tbsps. fresh basil
- 1 tsp. thyme
- 1 tsp. red pepper flakes
- 1 small onion, sliced
- 3 garlic cloves, minced
- 1 tbsp. olive oil
- 1 tsp. oregano
- 2 cups of water
- Salt and black pepper, to taste

DIRECTIONS:

1. Press Sauté and add oil, garlic, and onions in the pot. Cook for 4 minutes. Add red pepper flakes, oregano, basil, thyme, salt, and pepper.
2. Sauté for 1 minute and add tomatoes, carrots, water, and beans. Cover and cook on High for 40 minutes. Open and serve.

Nutrition: *calories 304, fat 10.3, fiber 5.4, carbs 46.8, protein 8.4*

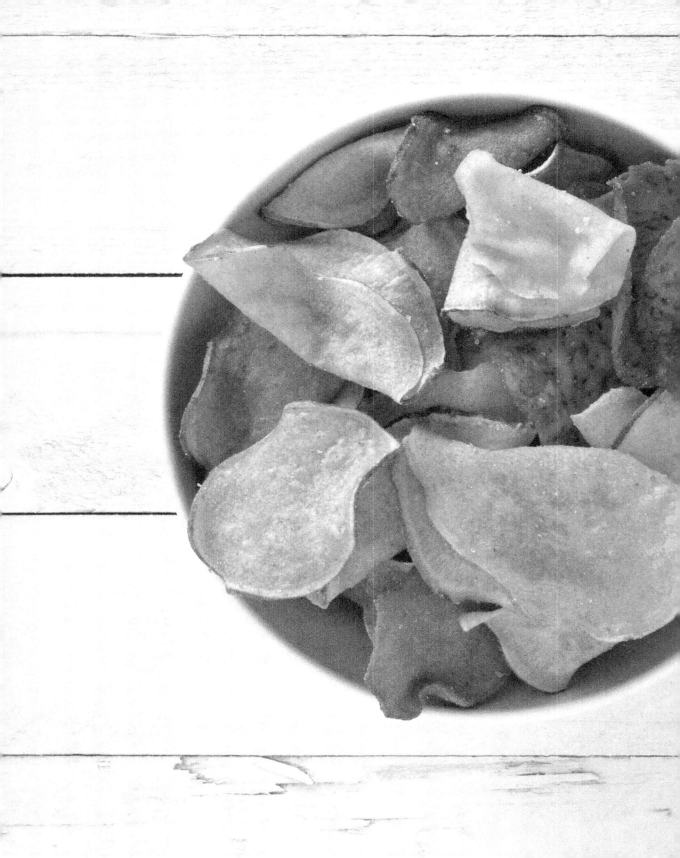

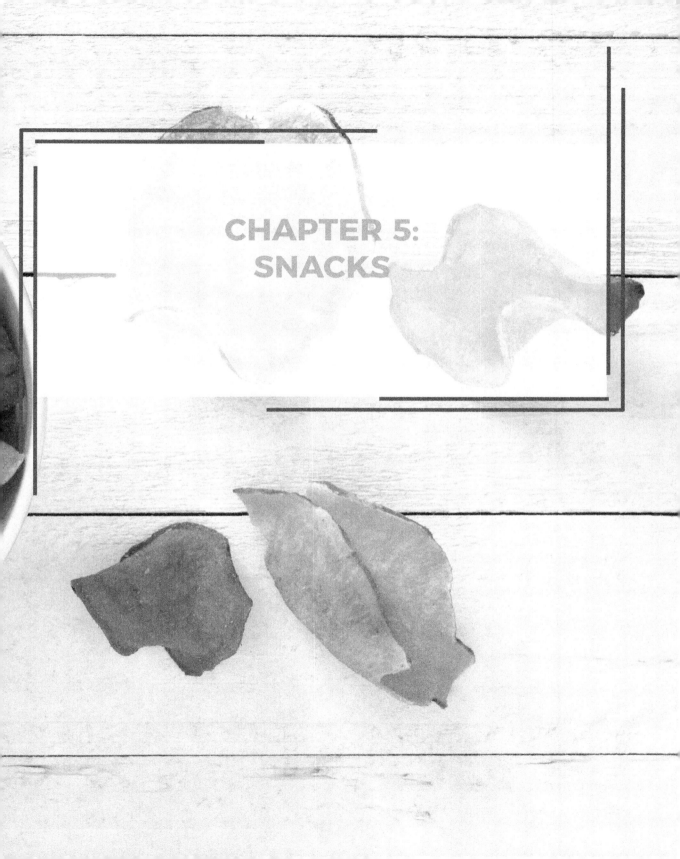

CHAPTER 5:
SNACKS

Preparation Time: 10 minutes
Cooking Time: 8 hours
Servings: 8

61. Green Bean Fries

INGREDIENTS:

- 1/3 cup avocado oil
- 5 pounds green beans, trimmed
- Salt and black pepper to the taste
- 1 teaspoon garlic powder
- 1 teaspoon onion powder
- 1 teaspoon turmeric powder
- 1 teaspoon oregano, dried
- 1 teaspoon mint, dried

DIRECTIONS:

1. In a bowl, mix the green beans with the oil, salt, pepper and the other ingredients and toss well.
2. Put the green beans in your dehydrator and dry them for 8 hours at 135 degrees. Serve cold as a snack.

Nutrition: *calories 100, fat 12, fiber 4, carbs 8, protein 5*

Preparation Time: 5 minutes
Cooking Time: 5 minutes
Servings: 5

62. Spiced Popcorn

INGREDIENTS:

- ½ cup corn kernels
- 4 tablespoons extra virgin olive oil
- ¼ cup za'atar spice
- A pinch of salt

DIRECTIONS:

1. Inside a bowl, mix the corn using the oil, za'at-ar, and salt and toss well.
2. Warm-up a pan over medium heat, add the corn, cook for 5 minutes until you get the popcorn and serve as a snack.

Nutrition: *Calories- 131, Fat- 5, Fiber- 4, Carbs- 7, Protein- 4*

Preparation Time: 5 minutes
Cooking Time: 0 minutes
Servings: 6

63. Mandarin Ambrosia

INGREDIENTS:

- ½ cup coconut cream, chilled in the refrigerator overnight
- 3 cups vegan mini marshmallows
- 1 cup shredded unsweetened coconut
- 3 small tangerines, peeled and segmented
- ½ cup sour cream

DIRECTIONS:

1. In a large bowl, beat the cold coconut cream until it forms stiff peaks.
2. Stir in the marshmallows, coconut, tangerine segments, and sour cream until well mixed.
3. Place it in the refrigerator for 3 hours before serving.

Nutrition: *Calories: 285 Total Fat: 22g Saturated Fat: 19g Protein: 4g Cholesterol: 6mg Sodium: 13mg Carbohydrates: 27g Fiber: 3g*

Preparation Time: 5 minutes
Cooking Time: 20 minutes
Servings: 6

64. Coconut-Quinoa Pudding

INGREDIENTS:

- 2 cups almond milk
- 1½ cups quinoa
- 1 cup light coconut milk
- ½ cup maple syrup
- Pinch salt
- 1 teaspoon pure vanilla extract

DIRECTIONS:

1. Heat the almond milk, quinoa, coconut milk, maple syrup, salt, and vanilla over medium-high heat in a large saucepan.
2. Bring the quinoa mixture to a boil and then reduce the heat to low.
3. Simmer until the quinoa is tender, stirring frequently, about 20 minutes.
4. Remove the pudding from the heat.
5. Serve warm.
6. Flavor Boost: If you are a chocolate enthusiast, stir 1 tablespoon of good-quality unsweetened cocoa powder into the almond milk and coconut milk before you combine the liquids with the other ingredients in step 1. This way you can remove any lumps in the cocoa powder before you add the quinoa. Increase the maple syrup to ¾ cup to offset the bitterness of the powder.

Nutrition: *Calories: 249 Total Fat: 6g Protein: 6g Cholesterol: 0mg Sodium: 161mg Carbohydrates: 42g Fiber: 3g*

Preparation Time: 5 minutes
Cooking Time: 20 minutes
Servings: 4

65. Stuffed Pears with Hazelnuts

INGREDIENTS:

- 1 tablespoon butter
- 2 ripe pears, cored and hollowed out with a spoon
- ½ cup water
- 8 tablespoons goat cheese
- 2 tablespoons honey
- ¼ cup roughly chopped hazelnuts

DIRECTIONS:

1. Preheat the oven to 350°f.
2. Melt the butter using a skillet on a medium heat.
3. Place the pears in the skillet, skin-side up, and lightly brown them, about 2 minutes.
4. Place the pears in an 8-by-8-inch square baking dish, hollow-side up, and pour water into the baking dish, make sure not to get any in the hollow part of the pears.
5. Roast the pears until softened, about 10 minutes. Remove the pears from the oven.
6. Using a small bowl, mix goat cheese, honey, and hazelnuts.
7. Divide the goat cheese mixture evenly between the pear halves and put them back in the oven for 5 minutes. Serve warm.

Nutrition: *Calories: 185 Total Fat: 9g Protein: 4g Cholesterol: 14mg Sodium: 75mg Carbohydrates: 26g Fiber: 4g*

Preparation Time: 10 minutes
Cooking Time: 2 minutes
Servings: 4

66. Buttermilk Panna Cotta with Mango

INGREDIENTS:

- ½ cup full-fat coconut milk
- 1½ teaspoons agar-agar
- 1½ cups buttermilk
- ¼ cup honey
- 2 cups roughly chopped fresh mango

DIRECTIONS:

1. Pour coconut milk into a saucepan, then sprinkle the agar-agar over it and let the coconut milk stand for 5 minutes.
2. Put the saucepan over medium-low heat until the agar-agar is dissolved, about 2 minutes.
3. Add the buttermilk and honey and stir to combine.
4. Pour the panna cotta mixture into 4 (6-ounce) ramekins. Wrap it in plastic wrap, then refrigerate them for about 3 hours, or until set.
5. Loosen the panna cotta by running a knife around the inside edges of the ramekins. Invert them onto serving plates.
6. Top with mango and serve.
7. Flavor Boost Vanilla beans add intense flavor and a pretty speckled appearance to this creamy dessert. Cut the vanilla bean in lengthwise and use a paring knife to scrape the seeds from one half into the buttermilk and honey in step 3. Wrap the other vanilla bean half in plastic and store in the fridge to use in smoothies or another dessert.

Nutrition: *Calories: 226 Total Fat: 8g Protein: 6g Cholesterol: 4mg Sodium: 106mg Carbohydrates: 36g Fiber: 2g*

Preparation Time: 15 minutes
Cooking Time: 15 minutes
Servings: 4

67. Sweet Potato-Cinnamon Parfaits

INGREDIENTS:

- 2 sweet potatoes, cut into ½-inch chunks
- 1 cup coconut cream, chilled in the refrigerator overnight
- ¼ cup maple syrup
- ¼ teaspoon ground cinnamon
- Pinch sea salt
- ½ cup roughly chopped hazelnuts

DIRECTIONS:

1. Get a large saucepan, then put the sweet potatoes. Fill the pan with water until the sweet potatoes are covered by about an inch. Boil over high heat and then reduce the heat and simmer until sweet potatoes are tender, about 15 minutes. Drain the water and mash sweet potatoes until smooth using a potato masher.
2. Transfer the sweet potatoes to a resealable container, and set it in the refrigerator until completely cooled, about 2 hours.
3. Whip the cold coconut cream until stiff peaks form using a large bowl.
4. Mix the sweet potatoes, maple syrup, cinnamon, and salt, then stir together in a bowl until smooth.
5. Fold half the whipped coconut cream into the sweet potato mixture, keeping as much volume as possible.
6. Chill the sweet potato mixture in the refrigerator for 1 hour.
7. Spoon the sweet potato mixture into 4 bowls and divide the remaining whipped coconut cream between the bowls.
8. Top with hazelnuts before serving.
9. Flavor Boost Hazelnuts have a wonderful, almost buttery-sweet flavor that is enhanced when roasted. Place ½ cup whole hazelnuts on a baking sheet and roast them in a 300°F oven for 10 to 15 minutes. Wait until the nuts cool and rub them between your hands to remove the skins. Chop and store the nuts in a sealed container in the cupboard for up to 1 week.

Nutrition: *Calories: 296 Total Fat: 12g Protein: 2g Cholesterol: 0mg Sodium: 70mg Carbohydrates: 41g Fiber: 1g*

Preparation Time: 5 minutes
Cooking Time: 15 minutes
Servings: 4

68. Sun-dried Tomato Pesto Snapper

INGREDIENTS:

- 1 sweet onion, cut into ¼-inch slices
- 4 (5-ounce) snapper fillets
- Freshly ground black pepper, for seasoning
- ¼ cup sun-dried tomato pesto
- 2 tablespoons finely chopped fresh basil

DIRECTIONS:

1. Preheat the oven to 400°F. Put parchment paper in a baking dish and arrange the onion slices on the bottom.
2. Pat the snapper fillets dry with a paper towel and season them lightly with pepper.
3. Place the fillets on the onions and spread 1 tablespoon of pesto on each fillet.
4. Bake until the fish flakes easily with a fork, 12 to 15 minutes.
5. Serve topped with basil.

Nutrition: *Calories: 199 Total Fat: 3g Protein: 36g Cholesterol: 66mg Sodium: 119mg Carbohydrates: 3g Fiber: 1g*

Preparation Time: 5 minutes
Cooking Time: 20 minutes
Servings: 4

69. Trout-Cilantro Packets

INGREDIENTS:

- 4 cups cauliflower florets
- 2 red bell peppers
- 2 cups snow peas, stringed
- 4 (5-ounce) trout fillets
- Sea salt, for seasoning
- Freshly ground black pepper, for seasoning
- 2 tablespoons olive oil
- 2 tablespoons finely chopped cilantro

DIRECTIONS:

1. Preheat the oven to 400°F.
2. Prepare four pieces of aluminum foil, each 12 inches square.
3. Evenly divide the cauliflower, bell peppers, and snow peas between the pieces of foil.
4. Pat dry the trout fillets with paper towels. Season them with salt and pepper.
5. Place a fillet on each foil square and drizzle the olive oil over the fish.
6. Fold the foil up to form tightly sealed packets and put them on a baking sheet.
7. Bake until cooked for about 20 minutes.
8. Serve topped with cilantro.

Nutrition: *Calories: 398 Total Fat: 23g Saturated Fat: 5g Protein: 35g Cholesterol: 80mg Sodium: 153mg Carbohydrates: 16g Fiber: 6g*

Preparation Time: **9 hours**
Cooking Time: **0 minute**
Serving: **8**

70.No Bake Mango Cheesecake

INGREDIENTS

- For the base
- 2 cups walnuts
- 3 tbsp coconut oil
- 3 tbsp shredded coconut
- 3 tbsp coconut nectar
- 1/8 tbsp salt
- For filling
- 2 cups brazil nuts
- 1 cup chopped zucchini
- 1/4 cup melted coconut oil
- 1/2 cup organic coconut nectar
- 1/2 tbsp vanilla powder
- 1/8 tbsp salt

DIRECTIONS:

1. Fit an S-blade in your food processor. Add walnuts and process into a fine meal. Add all the remaining base ingredients and process into a pliable dough that is slightly moist.
2. Line a baking tin with a parchment paper and add the walnut meal. place the tin in a freezer and freeze for about 30 minutes. In the meantime, process the nuts into your food processor on high speed until a fine meal.
3. Add all other filling ingredients and process until formation of a creamy consistency. Pour the filling into the baking tin and freeze for about 1 hour for the top layer to evenly spread. Now process the mango chunks until a smooth consistency.
4. Pour the mango puree over the filling. Now freeze the cheesecake for about 8 hours or overnight. Serve and enjoy.

Nutrition: *calories 354, fat 14g, fiber 2g, carbs 16g, protein 26g*

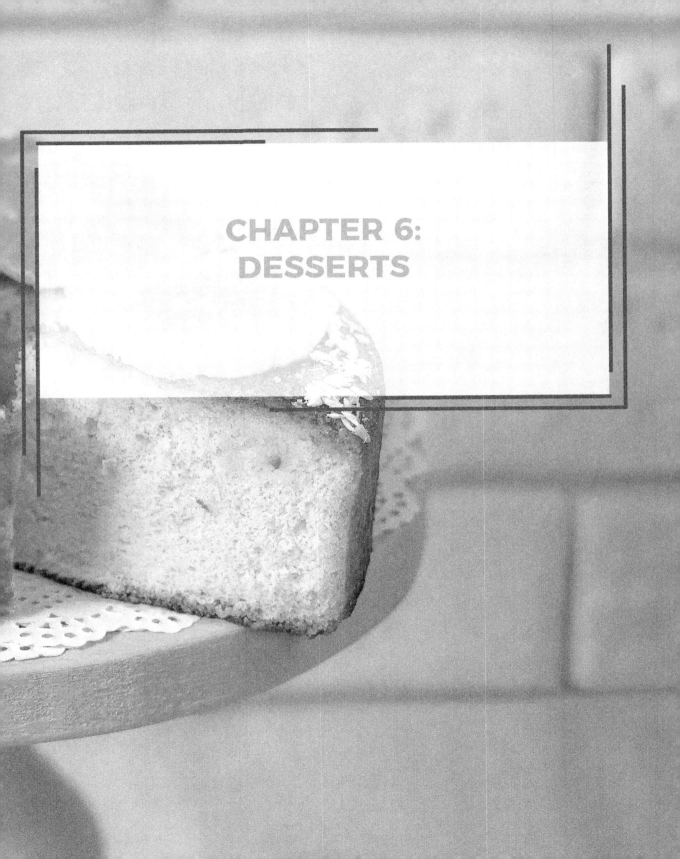

CHAPTER 6: DESSERTS

Preparation Time: 5 minutes
Cooking Time: 20 minutes
Serving: 1

71. Vegan Mango Ice Cream with Brazil Nuts

INGREDIENTS

- 4 ripe peeled mangoes, chopped
- 3/4 cups coconut milk
- 3-4 tbsp crushed Brazil nuts

DIRECTIONS:

1. Prepare your ice cream maker. Blend the mangoes until smooth and pour the puree into the ice cream maker bowl. Process milk in a blender a few times and pour into the bowl with mangoes.
2. Turn on the ice cream maker for about 10 minutes until a little thickening. Add a few Brazil nuts and reserving a few to garnish. Scoop the ice cream into an ice cream container then freeze for a few hours to solidify. Top with reserved Brazil nuts and serve.

Nutrition: *calories 354, fat 14, fiber 2, carbs 16, protein 26*

Preparation Time: 10 minutes
Cooking Time: 0 minute
Serving: 4

72. Watermelon and Bell Pepper Slush

INGREDIENTS

- 3 cups seeded watermelon, cubed
- 3 cups ice
- 1/2 seeded red bell pepper, coarsely chopped
- 1 spring fresh apple mint

DIRECTIONS:

1. Place watermelon, ice and pepper in a blender then blend until all ice is crushed and a slushy drink.
2. Transfer into glasses then garnish each with apple mint leaves. You can store for up to 2 days in a refrigerator. Serve and enjoy.

Nutrition: *calories 415, fat 35, fiber 2, carbs 8, protein 20*

Preparation Time: **5 minutes**
Cooking Time: **12 minutes**
Serving: **32**

73. Blackberry Jam

INGREDIENTS

- 3, 6-oz, package fresh berries, rinsed
- 3 tbsp agave nectar
- 1 tbsp key lime, squeezed juice
- 1/4 cup + 2 tbsp Sea moss gel

DIRECTIONS:

1. Place the berries into a pot, medium, over medium-high heat stirring until liquid starts to release and until they begin to break down. Stir in all other ingredients over about 1-2 minutes over low-medium heat until it starts to thicken.
2. Remove and cool for about 15 minutes. Serve with pancakes, waffles or toast.

Nutrition: *calories 210, fat 8, fiber 2, carbs 8, protein 7*

Preparation Time: **5 minutes**
Cooking Time: **0 minute**
Serving: **2**

74. Kale Berry Delight

INGREDIENTS

- 1 cup mixed berries
- 1 large apple
- 2 cups kale
- 1 cup water or coconut milk

DIRECTIONS:

1. Place berries, apple, kale, and water in a blender and blend until smooth. Serve and enjoy.

Nutrition: *calories 82, fat 4, fiber 2, carbs 14, protein 3*

75. Veggie Cakes

INGREDIENTS:

- Two teaspoons ginger, grated
- 1 cup yellow onion, chopped
- 1 cup mushrooms, minced
- 1 cup canned red lentils, drained
- ¼ cup veggie stock
- One sweet potato, chopped
- ¼ cup parsley, chopped
- ¼ cup hemp seeds
- One tablespoon curry powder
- ¼ cup cilantro, chopped
- A drizzle of olive oil
- 1 cup quick oats
- Two tablespoons rice flour

DIRECTIONS:

1. Warmth a pan with the oil on medium-high heat, add ginger, onion, and mushrooms, stir, and cook for 2-3 minutes.
2. Add lentils, potato, and stock, stir, cook for 5-6 minutes, take off heat, cool the whole mixture, and mash it with a fork.
3. Add parsley, cilantro, hemp, oats, curry powder, and rice flour, stir well and shape medium cakes out of this mix.
4. Place veggie cakes in your air fryer's basket and cook at 3750 F for 10 minutes, flipping them halfway.
5. Serve.
6. Enjoy!

Nutrition: *Calories: 212, Fat: 4 grams, Net Carbs: 8 grams, Protein: 10 grams*

76. Cinnamon Coconut Chips

INGREDIENTS:

- ¼ cup coconut chips, unsweetened
- ¼ teaspoon of sea salt
- ¼ cup cinnamon

DIRECTIONS:

1. Add cinnamon and salt in a mixing bowl and set aside. Heat a pan over medium heat for 2 minutes.
2. Place the coconut chips in the hot pan and stir until coconut chips crisp and lightly brown.
3. Toss toasted coconut chips with cinnamon and salt.
4. Serve and enjoy!

Nutrition: *Calories: 228, Fat: 21 grams, Net Carbs: 7.8 grams, Protein: 1.9 grams*

Preparation Time: 10 Minutes
Cooking Time: 20 Minutes
Servings: 4

77. Chocolate Brownies

INGREDIENTS

- Two tablespoons cocoa powder
- One scoop protein powder
- 1 cup bananas, over-ripe
- ½ cup almond butter, melted

DIRECTIONS:

1. Preheat the oven to 350 F.
2. Spray the brownie pan with cooking spray.
3. Add the real ingredients in your blender and blend until smooth.
4. Pour the batter into the prepared pan.
5. Put in the oven for 20 minutes.
6. Serve and enjoy!

Nutrition: *Calories: 82, Fat: 2.1 grams, Net Carbs: 11.4 grams, Protein: 6.9 grams*

Preparation Time: 30 Minutes
Cooking Time: 1 Hour and 15 Minutes
Servings:

78. The Keto Lovers "Magical" Grain-Free Granola

INGREDIENTS:

- ½ cup of raw sunflower seeds
- ½ cup of raw hemp hearts
- ½ cup of flaxseeds
- ¼ cup of chia seeds
- Two tablespoons of Psyllium Husk powder
- One tablespoon of cinnamon
- Stevia
- ½ teaspoon of baking powder
- ½ teaspoon of salt
- 1 cup of water

DIRECTIONS:

1. Preheat your oven to 300 F. Make sure to line a baking page with a parchment piece.
2. Take your food processor and grind all the seeds.
3. Add the dry ingredients and mix well.
4. Stir in water until fully incorporated.
5. Let the mixture sit for a while. Wait until it thickens up.
6. Spread the mixture evenly-giving a thickness of about ¼ inch.
7. Bake for 45 minutes.
8. Break apart the granola and keep baking for another 30 minutes until the pieces are crunchy.
9. Remove and allow them to cool.
10.   Enjoy!

Nutrition: *Calories: 292, Fat: 25 grams, Net Carbs: 12 grams, Protein: 8 grams*

Preparation Time: 10 minutes
Cooking Time: 20 minutes
Servings: 6

79. Rhubarb and Strawberry Dessert

INGREDIENTS:

- 3 tbsp. stevia
- 1 pound strawberries, halved
- 1/3 cup water
- 2 pounds rhubarb, roughly chopped
- A few mint leaves, chopped

DIRECTION

1. In your instant pot, mix water with rhubarb, stevia and strawberries.
2. Sit a bit, cover and cook on High for 10 minutes.
3. Add the mint leaves. Leave aside for a few minutes.
4. Divide into cups. Serve and enjoy!

Nutrition: *calories 127, fat 3.3, fiber 2.8, carbs 22.5, protein 3.2*

Prep Time: 10 minutes
Cooking Time: 50 minutes
Servings: 9

80. Lemon Cake

INGREDIENTS:

- 1 ½ cup white whole-wheat flour
- 1 ½ teaspoon baking powder
- 2 tablespoons almond flour
- 1 lemon, zested
- ¼ teaspoon baking soda
- 1/8 teaspoon turmeric powder
- 1/3 teaspoon salt
- ¼ teaspoon vanilla extract, unsweetened
- 1/3 cup lemon juice
- ½ cup maple syrup
- ¼ cup olive oil
- ¼ cup of water
- For the Frosting:
- 1 tablespoon lemon juice
- 1/8 teaspoon salt
- ¼ cup maple syrup
- 2 tablespoons powdered sugar
- 6 ounces vegan cream cheese, softened

DIRECTIONS:

1. Switch on the oven, then set it to 350 degrees F and let it preheat.
2. Take a large bowl, pour in water, lemon juice, and oil, add vanilla extract and maple syrup, and whisk until blended.
3. Whisk in flour, ¼ cup at a time, until smooth, and then whisk in almond flour, salt, turmeric, lemon zest, baking soda, and powder until well combined.
4. Take a loaf pan, grease it with oil, spoon prepared batter in it, and then bake for 50 minutes.
5. Meanwhile, prepare the frosting and for this, take a small bowl, place all of its ingredients in it, whisk until smooth, and then let it chill until required.
6. When the cake has cooked, let it cool for 10 minutes in its pan and then let it cool completely on the wire rack.
7. Spread the prepared frosting on top of the cake, slice the cake, and then serve.

Nutrition: *Calories: 275 Cal; Fat: 12 g; Protein: 3 g; Carbs: 38 g; Fiber: 1 g*

Preparation Time: 10 minutes
Cooking Time: 0 minutes
Servings: 8

81. Creamy Peach Ice Pops

INGREDIENTS

- 1 (14-ounce) can light coconut milk
- 2 peaches, peeled, pitted, and roughly chopped
- ¼ cup honey
- Pinch cinnamon

DIRECTIONS:

1. In a blender, blend the coconut milk, peaches, honey, and cinnamon until smooth.
2. Pour the mixture into ice pop molds and freeze for about 5 hours.
3. Can stored for a week in the freezer using plastic wrap over the open tops of the molds.
4. Substitution Tip: You can create a staggering variety of wonderful flavors by swapping out the peaches for other ingredients—you'll need about 3 cups total. Try peeled plums, watermelon, cantaloupe, berries, sweet potato, mango, pineapple, and papaya in any combination or alone. Add an amount of honey, depending on the sweetness of the base ingredient.

Nutrition: *Calories: 79 Total Fat: 3g Protein: 0g Cholesterol: 0mg Sodium: 4mg Carbohydrates: 13g Fiber: 1g*

Preparation Time: 15 minutes
Cooking Time: 0 minutes
Servings: 8

82. Melon-Lime Sorbet

INGREDIENTS

- 1 small honeydew melon, cut into 1-inch chunks
- 1 small cantaloupe, cut into 1-inch chunks
- 2 tablespoons honey
- 2 tablespoons freshly squeezed lime juice
- Pinch cinnamon
- Water as needed

DIRECTIONS:

1. Spread the honeydew and cantaloupe out on a baking sheet lined with parchment paper, then place in the freezer for up to 4 to 6 hours or until frozen.
2. In a food processor, add the frozen melon chunks and the honey, lime juice, and cinnamon.
3. Pulse and wait until smooth, add water (a tablespoon at a time) if needed to purée the melon.
4. Transfer the mixture to a container that is resalable and place in the freezer until set, about 30 minutes.
5. Substitution Tip: Almost any fruit will work in this recipe. You can try watermelon, peaches, plums, mangos, or berries. Some fruit has more water in it than others, so if you're using produce that's less juicy, add extra water or apple juice to create a smooth purée.

Nutrition: *Calories: 97 Total Fat: 0g Protein: 2g Cholesterol: 0mg Sodium: 39mg Carbohydrates: 25g Fiber: 2g*

Prep Time: 10 minutes
Cooking Time: 30 minutes
Yields: 12

83. Banana Muffins

INGREDIENTS:

- 1 ½ cups mashed banana
- 1 ½ cups and 2 tablespoons white whole-wheat flour, divided
- ¼ cup of coconut sugar
- ¾ cup rolled oats, divided
- 1 teaspoon ginger powder
- 1 tablespoon ground cinnamon, divided
- 2 teaspoons baking powder
- ½ teaspoon salt
- 1 teaspoon baking soda
- 1 tablespoon vanilla extract, un-sweetened
- ½ cup maple syrup
- 1 tablespoon rum
- ½ cup of coconut oil

DIRECTIONS:

1. Switch on the oven, then set it to 350 degrees F and let it preheat.
2. Meanwhile, take a medium bowl, place 1 ½ cup flour in it, add ½ cup oars, ginger, baking powder and soda, salt, and 2 teaspoons cinnamon and then stir until mixed.
3. Place ¼ cup of coconut oil in a heatproof bowl, melt it in the microwave oven and then whisk in maple syrup until combined.
4. Add mashed banana along with rum and vanilla, stir until combined, and then whisk this mixture into the flour mixture until smooth batter comes together.
5. Take a separate medium bowl, place remaining oats and flour in it, add cinnamon, coconut sugar, and coconut oil and then stir with a fork until crumbly mixture comes together.
6. Take a 12-cups muffin pan, fill evenly with prepared batter, top with oats mixture, and then bake for 30 minutes until firm and the top turn golden brown.
7. When done, let the muffins cool for 5 minutes in its pan and then cool the muffins completely before serving.

Nutrition: *Calories: 240 Cal; Fat: 9.3 g; Protein: 2.6 g; Carbs: 35.4 g; Fiber: 2 g*

Preparation Time: 30 minutes
Cooking Time: 0 minutes
Servings: 9

84. No-Bake Cookies

INGREDIENTS:

- 1 cup rolled oats
- ¼ cup of cocoa powder
- 1/8 teaspoon salt
- 1 teaspoon vanilla extract, un-sweetened
- ¼ cup and 2 tablespoons peanut butter, divided
- 6 tablespoons coconut oil, divided
- ¼ cup and 1 tablespoon maple syrup, divided

DIRECTIONS:

1. Take a small saucepan, place it over low heat, add 5 tablespoons of coconut oil and then let it melt.
2. Whisk in 2 tablespoons peanut butter, salt, 1 teaspoon vanilla extract, and ¼ cup each of cocoa powder and maple syrup, and then whisk until well combined.
3. Remove pan from heat, stir in oats and then spoon the mixture evenly into 9 cups of a muffin pan.
4. Wipe clean the pan, return it over low heat, add remaining coconut oil, maple syrup, and peanut butter, stir until combined, and then cook for 2 minutes until thoroughly warmed.
5. Drizzle the peanut butter sauce over the oat mixture in the muffin pan and then let it freeze for 20 minutes or more until set.
6. Serve straight away.

Nutrition: *Calories: 213 Cal; Fat: 14.8 g; Protein: 4 g; Carbs: 17.3 g; Fiber: 2.1 g*

Prep Time: 40 minutes
Cooking Time: 8 minutes
Servings: 8

85. Peanut Butter and Oat Bars

INGREDIENTS:

- 1 cup rolled oats
- 1/8 teaspoon salt
- ¼ cup chocolate chips, vegan
- ¼ cup maple syrup
- 1 cup peanut butter

Nutrition: *Calories: 274 Cal; Fat: 17 g; Protein: 10 g; Carbs: 19 g; Fiber: 3 g*

DIRECTIONS:

1. Take a medium saucepan, place it over medium heat, add peanut butter, salt, and maple syrup and then whisk until combined and thickened; this will take 5 minutes.
2. Remove pan from heat, place oats in a bowl, pour peanut butter mixture on it and then stir until well combined.
3. Take an 8-by-6 inches baking dish, line it with a parchment sheet, spoon the oats mixture in it, and then spread evenly, pressing the mixture into the dish.
4. Sprinkle the chocolate chips on top, press them into the bar mixture and then let the mixture rest in the refrigerator for 30 minutes or more until set.
5. When ready to eat, cut the bar mixture into even size pieces and then serve.

Preparation Time: 5 minutes
Cooking Time: 20 minutes
Servings: 4

86. Baked Apples

INGREDIENTS:

- 6 medium apples, peeled, cut into chunks
- 1 teaspoon ground cinnamon
- 2 tablespoons melted coconut oil

DIRECTIONS:

1. Switch on the oven, then set it to 350 degrees F and let it preheat.
2. Take a medium baking dish, and then spread apple pieces in it.
3. Take a small bowl, place coconut oil in it, stir in cinnamon, drizzle this mixture over apples and then toss until coated.
4. Place the baking dish into the oven and then bake for 20 minutes or more until apples turn soft, stirring halfway.
5. Serve straight away.

Nutrition: *Calories: 170 Cal; Fat: 3.8 g; Protein: 0.5 g; Carbs: 31 g; Fiber: 5.5 g*

Preparation Time: 10 Minutes
Cooking Time: 3-4 Hours to Freeze
Servings: 4-5

87. Keto Ice Cream

INGREDIENTS:

- 1 ½ teaspoon of natural vanilla extract
- 1/8 teaspoon of salt
- 1/3 cup of erythritol
- 2 cups of artificial coconut milk, full fat

DIRECTIONS:

1. Stir together the vanilla extract, salt, sweetener, and milk.
2. If you do not come up with an ice cream machine, freeze the mixture in ice cube trays, then use a high-speed blender to blend the frozen cubes or thaw them enough to meld in a regular blender or food processor.
3. If you have an ice cream machine, just blend according to the manufacturer's directions.
4. Eat as it is or freeze for a firmer texture.

Nutrition: *Calories: 184, Fat: 19.1 grams, Net Carbs: 4.4 grams, Protein: 1.8 grams*

Preparation Time: 10 Minutes
Cooking Time: 4 Hours
Servings: 6

88. Apple Mix

INGREDIENTS:

- Six apples, cored, peeled, and sliced
- 1½ cups almond flour
- Cooking spray
- 1 cup of coconut sugar
- One tablespoon cinnamon powder
- ¾ cup cashew butter, melted

DIRECTIONS:

1. Add apple slices to your slow cooker after you have greased it with cooking spray.
2. Add flour, sugar, cinnamon, and coconut butter, stir gently, cover, cook on High for 4 hours, divide into bowls and serve cold.
3. Enjoy!

Nutrition: *Calories: 200, Fat: 5 grams, Net Carbs: 8 grams, Protein: 4 grams*

Preparation Time: **17 Minutes**
Cooking Time: **2-3 Hours to Freeze**
Servings: **8**

89. Almond Butter Fudge

INGREDIENTS:

- 2 ½ tablespoons coconut oil
- 2 ½ tablespoons honey
- ½ cup almond butter

DIRECTIONS:

1. In a saucepan, pour almond butter then add coconut oil warm for 2 minutes or until melted.
2. Add honey and stir.
3. Pour the mixture into a candy container and store it in the fridge until set.
4. Serve and enjoy!

Nutrition: *Calories: 63, Fat: 4.8 grams, Net Carbs: 5.6 grams, Protein: 0.2 grams*

Preparation Time: **20 Minutes**
Cooking Time: **1 Hour and 20 Minutes**
Servings: **12**

90. The Vegan Pumpkin Spicy Fat Bombs

INGREDIENTS:

- ¾ cup of pumpkin puree
- ¼ cup of hemp seeds
- ½ cup of coconut oil
- Two teaspoons of pumpkin pie spice
- One teaspoon of vanilla extract
- Liquid Stevia

DIRECTIONS:

1. Take a blender and add together all the ingredients.
2. Blend them well and portion the mixture out into silicon molds.
3. Allow them to chill and enjoy!

Nutrition: *Calories: 103, Fat: 10 grams, Net Carbs: 2 grams, Protein: 1 gram*

Preparation Time: 25 Minutes
Cooking Time: 5 Hours and 10 Minutes
Servings: 4

91. Orange Cake

INGREDIENTS:

- Cooking spray
- One teaspoon baking powder
- 1 cup almond flour
- 1 cup of coconut sugar
- ½ teaspoon cinnamon powder
- Three tablespoons coconut oil, melted
- ½ cup almond milk
- ½ cup pecans, chopped
- ¾ cup of water
- ½ cup raisins
- ½ cup orange peel, grated
- ¾ cup of orange juice

DIRECTIONS:

1. In a bowl, mix flour with half of the sugar, baking powder, cinnamon, two tablespoons oil, milk, pecans, and raisins, stir and pour this in your slow cooker after you have sprayed it with cooking spray.
2. Warm a small pan over medium heat. Add water, orange juice, orange peel, the rest of the oil, and the remainder of the sugar, stir, bring to a boil, pour over the blend in the slow cooker, cover, and cook on Low for 5 hours.
3. Divide into dessert bowls and serve cold.
4. Enjoy!

Nutrition: *Calories: 182, Fat: 3 grams Net Carbs: 4 grams, Protein: 3 grams*

Preparation Time: 10 minutes
Cooking Time: 10 minutes
Servings: 4

92. Vanilla Peach Mix

INGREDIENTS:

- 4 cups water
- 3 peaches, chopped
- 2 cups rolled oats
- 1 teaspoon vanilla extract
- 2 tablespoons flax meal

DIRECTIONS:

1. In a pan, combine the peaches with the water and the other ingredients, stir, bring to a simmer over medium heat, cook for 10 minutes, divide into bowls and serve.

Nutrition: *calories 161, fat 3, fiber 3, carbs 7, protein 5*

Preparation Time: 10 minutes
Cooking Time: 0 minutes
Servings: 4

93. Ginger Ice Cream

INGREDIENTS:

- 4 cups coconut milk
- 2 tablespoons fresh grated ginger
- 3 tablespoons stevia
- 2 teaspoons ground turmeric
- ½ teaspoon ground cinnamon
- 1 teaspoon ground cardamom
- 1 teaspoon vanilla extract

DIRECTIONS:

1. In a blender, combine the coconut milk with the ginger and the other ingredients and blend well.
2. Transfer the ice cream to an ice cream machine and process for 30 minutes, then freeze for another 3 hours before serving.

Nutrition: *calories 200, fat 4.4, fiber 9, carbs 5.2, protein 7*

Preparation Time: 10 minutes.
Cooking Time: 1 hour
Servings: 6

94. Shortbread Cookies

INGREDIENTS:

- 2 1/2 cups coconut flour
- 6 tablespoons walnut butter
- 1/2 cup erythritol
- 1 teaspoon vanilla essence

DIRECTIONS:

1. Preheat your oven to 350 degrees F.
2. Layer a cookie sheet with parchment paper.
3. Beat butter with erythritol until fluffy.
4. Stir in vanilla essence and coconut flour. Mix well until crumbly.
5. Spoon out a tablespoon of cookie dough onto the cookie sheet.
6. Add more dough to make as many cookies.
7. Bake for 15 minutes until brown.
8. Serve.

Nutrition: *Calories: 288 Fat: 25.3g. Carbs: 9.6g. Protein: 7.6g. Fiber: 3.8g.*

Preparation Time: 10 minutes.
Cooking Time: 15 minutes.
Servings: 4

95. Coconut Chip Cookies

INGREDIENTS:

- 1 cup coconut flour
- ½ cup cacao nibs
- ½ cup coconut flakes, unsweetened
- 1/3 cup erythritol
- ½ cup walnut butter
- ¼ cup walnut butter, melted
- ¼ cup coconut milk
- Stevia, to taste
- ¼ teaspoon sea salt

DIRECTIONS:

1. Preheat your oven to 350 degrees F.
2. Layer a cookie sheet with parchment paper.
3. Add and combine all the dry ingredients in a glass bowl.
4. Whisk in butter, coconut milk, vanilla essence, stevia, and walnut butter.
5. Beat well then stir in the dry mixture. Mix well.
6. Spoon out a tablespoon of cookie dough on the cookie sheet.
7. Add more dough to make as many as 16 cookies.
8. Flatten each cookie using your fingers.
9. Bake for 25 minutes until golden brown.
10. Let them sit for 15 minutes.
11. Serve.

Nutrition: *Calories: 192 Fat: 17.44g. Carbs: 2.2g. Protein: 4.7g. Fiber: 2.1g.*

Preparation Time: 5 minutes
Cooking Time: 2 hours
Servings: 2

96. Cinnamon Baked Apple Chips

INGREDIENTS:

- 1 teaspoon cinnamon
- 1-2 apples

DIRECTIONS:

1. Preheat your oven to 200 degrees Fahrenheit
2. Take a sharp knife and slice apples into thin slices
3. Discard seeds
4. Line a baking sheet with parchment paper and arrange apples on it
5. Make sure they do not overlap
6. Once done, sprinkle cinnamon over apples
7. Bake in the oven for 1 hour
8. Flip and bake for an hour more until no longer moist
9. Serve and enjoy!

Nutrition: *calories 82, fat 4, fiber 2, carbs 14, protein 3*

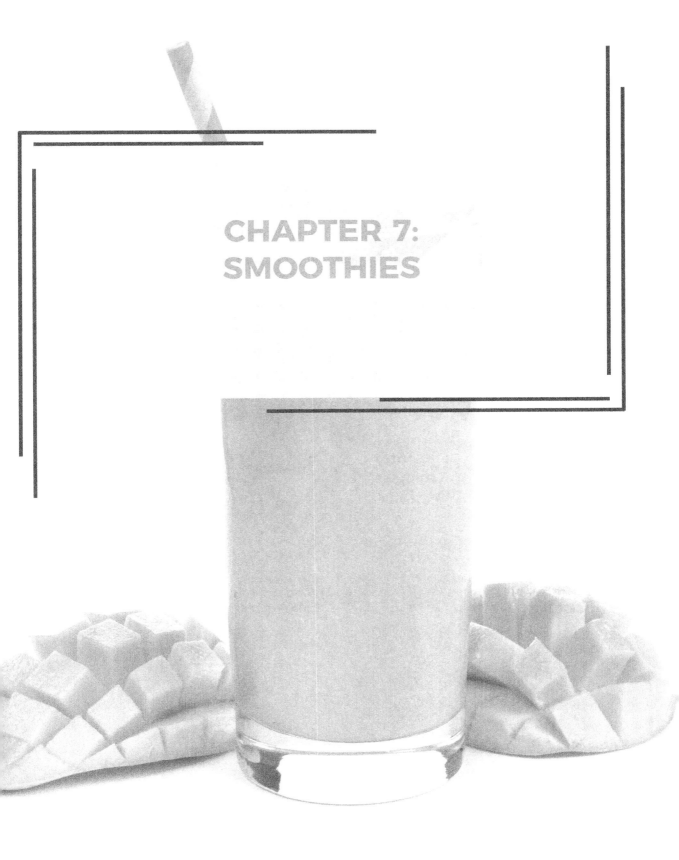

CHAPTER 7:
SMOOTHIES

Preparation Time: 5 minutes
Cooking Time: 0 minutes
Servings: 2

97. Piña Colada Smoothie Bowl

INGREDIENTS:

- 2 bananas, sliced and frozen
- 1 cup frozen mango chunks
- 1 (20-ounce) can pineapple chunks, drained
- 1 (14-ounce) can of full-fat coconut milk
- 1 teaspoon vanilla extract
- Water, for thinning (optional)
- Hemp seeds, for garnish
- Cashew butter, for garnish
- Chia seeds, for garnish (optional)
- Starfruit slices, for garnish (optional)
- Fresh pitted cherries for garnish (optional)

DIRECTIONS:

1. In a high-speed blender or food processor, combine the bananas, mango, pineapple, coconut milk, and vanilla. Blend until smooth.
2. This smoothie will be thick and may require several starts and stops to scrape the sides down. If it seems too thick, add water to thin.
3. Serve in a bowl topped with hemp seeds, cashew butter, chia seeds, starfruit, and cherries (if using). Enjoy as a refreshing drink instead of adding water.

Nutrition: *Calories: 678, Fat: 38g Protein: 5g, Carbohydrates: 89g*

Preparation Time: 5 minutes
Cooking Time: 0 minutes
Servings: 1

98. Beet Fruit Smoothie

INGREDIENTS:

- 1½ cups unsweetened plant-based milk
- 1 Granny Smith apple, peeled, cored, and chopped
- 1 cup chopped frozen beets
- 1 cup frozen blueberries
- ½ cup frozen cherries
- ¼-inch fresh ginger root, peeled

DIRECTIONS:

1. In a blender, combine all the ingredients and blend until smooth. Serve immediately or store in the freezer in a resealable jar.

Nutrition: *Calories: 324; Fat: 5g; Carbs: 70g; Protein: 5g; Fiber: 15g*

Preparation Time: 5 minutes
Cooking Time: 0 minutes
Servings: 2

99. Banana and Mango Smoothie Bowls

INGREDIENTS

- 2 bananas, sliced and frozen
- 1 cup frozen mango chunks
- 1 (20-ounce / 567-g) can pineapple chunks, drained
- 1 (14-ounce / 397-g) can full-fat coconut milk
- 1 teaspoon vanilla extract
- Water, for thinning (optional)
- Hemp seeds, for garnish
- Cashew butter, for garnish
- Chia seeds, for garnish (optional)
- Starfruit slices, for garnish (optional)
- Fresh pitted cherries, for garnish (optional)

DIRECTIONS:

1. In a high-speed blender or food processor, combine the bananas, mango, pineapple, coconut milk, and vanilla. Blend until smooth. This smoothie will be thick and may require several starts and stops to scrape the sides down. If it seems too thick, add water to thin.
2. Serve in a bowl topped with hemp seeds, cashew butter, chia seeds, starfruit, and cherries (if using). Enjoy as a refreshing drink instead by adding water.

Nutrition (1 smoothie): *Calories: 678; Fat: 38g; Carbs: 89g; Protein: 5g; Fiber: 8g*

Preparation Time: 10 minutes
Cooking Time: 0 minutes
Servings: 2

100. Mango Smoothie

INGREDIENTS:

- 1 cup mango, chopped
- 1 tablespoon stevia
- 1 teaspoon almond extract
- 1 cup pineapple, chopped
- 1 cup almond milk

DIRECTIONS:

1. In a blender, mix the mango with the stevia and the other ingredients, pulse and serve for breakfast.

Nutrition: *calories 122, fat 2, fiber 4, carbs 5.2, protein 6*

Preparation Time: 5 minutes
Cooking Time: 0 minutes
Servings: 1

101. Power Green Smoothie

INGREDIENTS:

- 3 cups fresh spinach
- 1½ cups frozen pineapple
- 1 cup unsweetened plant-based milk
- 1 cup fresh kale
- 1 Granny Smith apple, peeled, cored, and chopped
- ½ small avocado, pitted and peeled
- ½ teaspoon spirulina
- 1 tablespoon hemp seeds

DIRECTIONS:

1. In a blender, combine all the ingredients and blend until smooth. Serve immediately or store in the freezer in a resealable jar.

Nutrition: *Calories: 431; Fat: 16g; Carbs: 70g; Protein: 13g; Fiber: 17g*

Preparation Time: 5 minutes
Cooking Time: 0 minutes
Servings: 1

102. Pineapple Coconut Smoothie

INGREDIENTS:

- 2 cups frozen pineapple
- 1 banana
- 1¼ cups unsweetened coconut milk
- ¼ cup frozen coconut pieces
- ½ teaspoon ground flaxseed
- 1 teaspoon hemp seeds

DIRECTIONS:

1. In a blender, combine all the ingredients and blend until smooth. Serve immediately or store in the freezer in a resealable jar.

Nutrition: *Calories: 396; Fat: 14g; Carbs: 71g; Protein: 6g; Fiber: 11g*

Preparation Time: 5 minutes
Cooking Time: 0 minutes
Servings: 1

103. Berry Smoothie

INGREDIENTS:

- 1 banana
- 1¼ cups unsweetened plant-based milk
- ½ cup frozen strawberries
- ½ cup frozen blueberries
- ½ cup frozen raspberries
- 3 pitted Medjool dates
- 1 tablespoon hulled hemp seeds
- ½ tablespoon ground flaxseed
- 1 teaspoon ground chia seeds

DIRECTIONS:

1. In a blender, combine all the ingredients and blend until smooth. Serve immediately or store in the freezer in a resealable jar.

Nutrition: *Calories: 538; Fat: 11g; Carbs: 111g; Protein: 10g; Fiber: 21g*

Preparation Time: 5 minutes
Cooking Time: 0 minutes
Servings: 2

104. Chocolate Green Smoothie

INGREDIENTS:

- 6 ounces (170 g) greens (kale, collards, or spinach)
- 2 very ripe frozen bananas, halved
- 3 cups plant-based milk
- 2 tablespoons cocoa powder
- 1 teaspoon vanilla extract

DIRECTIONS:

1. In a blender, combine the greens, bananas, milk, cocoa powder, and vanilla. Blend on high for 1 to 2 minutes, or until the contents reach a smooth and creamy consistency, and serve.

Nutrition: *Calories: 225; Fat: 6g; Carbs: 42g; Protein: 6g; Fiber: 8g*

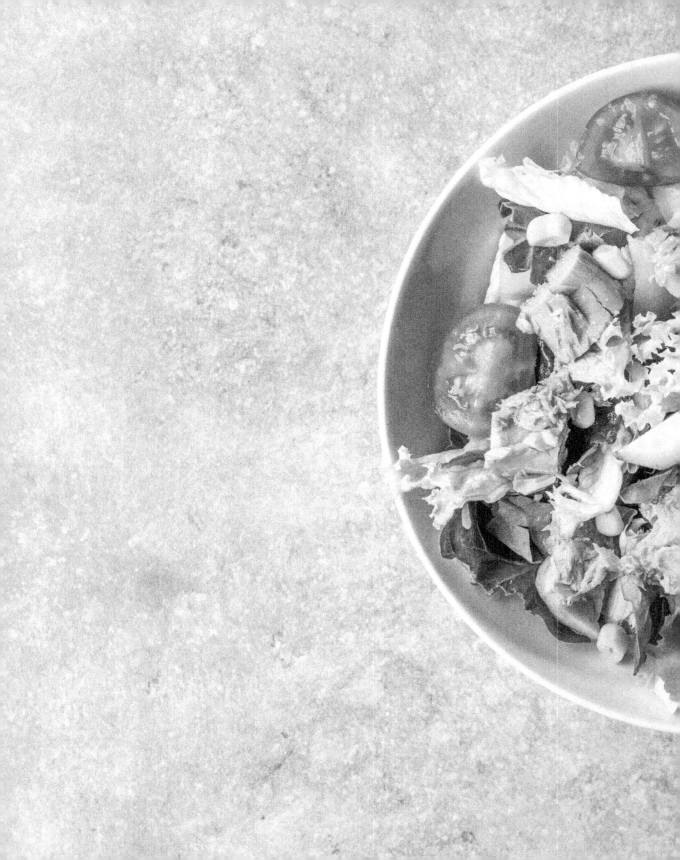

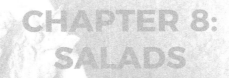

CHAPTER 8:
SALADS

Preparation Time: 10 minutes
Cooking Time: 40 minutes
Servings: 4

105. Caramelized Onion And Beet Salad

INGREDIENTS:

- 3 medium golden beets
- 2 cups sliced sweet or Vidalia onions
- 1 teaspoon extra-virgin olive oil or no-beef broth
- Pinch baking soda
- ¼ to ½ teaspoon salt, to taste
- 2 tablespoons unseasoned rice vinegar, white wine vinegar, or balsamic vinegar

Nutrition: *Calories: 104; Fat: 2g; Protein: 3g; Carbohydrates: 20g; Fiber: 4g; Sugar: 14g; Sodium: 303mg*

DIRECTIONS:

1. Preparing the Ingredients
2. Cut the greens off the beets, and scrub the beets.
3. In a large pot, place a steamer basket and fill the pot with 2 inches of water.
4. Add the beets, bring to boil, then reduce the heat to medium, cover, and steam for about 35 minutes until you can easily pierce the middle of the beets with a knife.
5. Meanwhile, in a large, dry skillet over medium heat, sauté the onions for 5 minutes while stirring frequently.
6. Add the olive oil and baking soda, then continuing cooking for 5 more minutes while stirring frequently. Stir in the salt before removing from the heat. Transfer to a large bowl and set aside.
7. Finish and Serve
8. When the beets have cooked through, drain and cool until easy to handle. Rub the beets in a paper towel to easily remove the skins. Cut into wedges, and transfer to the bowl with the onions. Drizzle the vinegar over everything and toss well.
9. Divide the beets evenly among 4 wide-mouth jars or storage containers. Let it cool before sealing the lids.

Preparation Time: 10 minutes
Cooking Time: 50 minutes
Servings: 4

106. Warm Lentil Salad with Red Wine Vinaigrette

INGREDIENTS:

- 1 teaspoon extra-virgin olive oil plus ¼ cup, divided, or 1 tablespoon vegetable broth or water
- 1 small onion, diced
- 1 garlic clove, minced
- 1 carrot, diced
- 1 cup lentils
- 1 tablespoon dried basil
- 1 tablespoon dried oregano
- 1 tablespoon red wine or balsamic vinegar (optional)
- 2 cups water
- ¼ cup red wine vinegar or balsamic vinegar
- 1 teaspoon sea salt
- 2 cups chopped Swiss chard
- 2 cups torn red leaf lettuce
- 4 tablespoons Cheesy Sprinkle

Nutrition: *Calories: 387; Total fat: 17g; Carbs: 42g; Fiber: 19g; Protein: 18g*

DIRECTIONS:

1. Preparing the Ingredients
2. Heat 1 teaspoon of the oil in a large pot on medium heat, then sauté the onion and garlic until they are translucent.
3. Add the carrot and sauté until it is slightly cooked. Stir in the lentils, basil, and oregano, then add the wine or balsamic vinegar (if using).
4. Pour the water into the pot and turn the heat up to high to bring to boil.
5. Turn the heat down to a simmer and let the lentils cook, uncovered, for 20-30 minutes until they are soft but not falling apart.
6. While the lentils are cooking, whisk together the red wine vinegar, olive oil, and salt in a small bowl and set aside. Once the lentils have cooked, drain any excess liquid and stir in most of the red wine vinegar dressing. Set a little bit of dressing aside. Add the Swiss chard to the pot and stir it into the lentils. Leave the heat on low and cook, stirring, for at least 10 minutes.
7. Finish and Serve
8. Toss the lettuce with the remaining dressing. Place some lettuce on a plate, and top with the lentil mixture. Finish the plate off with a little cheesy sprinkle and enjoy.

Preparation Time: 15 minutes
Cooking Time: 0 minutes
Servings: 4

107. Red Bean And Corn Salad

INGREDIENTS:

- ¼ cup Cashew Cream or other salad dressing
- 1 teaspoon chili powder
- 2 (14.5-ounce) cans kidney beans, rinsed and drained
- 2 cups frozen corn, thawed, or 2 cups canned corn, drained
- 1 cup cooked farro, barley, or rice (optional)
- 8 cups chopped romaine lettuce

DIRECTIONS:

1. Preparing the Ingredients
2. Line up 4 wide-mouth glass quart jars.
3. In a small bowl, whisk the cream and chili powder. Pour 1 tablespoon of cream into each jar. In each jar, add ¾ cup kidney beans, ½ cup corn, ¼ cup cooked farro (if using), and 2 cups romaine, punching it down to fit it into the jar. Close the lids tightly.

Per Serving: *Calories: 303; Fat: 9g; Protein: 14g; Carbohydrates: 45g; Fiber: 15g; Sugar: 6g; Sodium: 654mg*

Preparation Time: 10 minutes
Cooking Time: 0 minutes
Serving: 4

108. Tuna Salad

INGREDIENTS:

- 1/2 cup chopped celery
- 3 cups cooked chickpeas
- 1 tablespoon capers, chopped
- 2 tablespoons sweet pickle relish
- 1 tablespoon yellow mustard paste
- 2 tablespoons mayonnaise

DIRECTIONS:

1. Take a medium bowl, place chickpeas in it, add mustard and mayonnaise and mash by using a fork until peas are broken.
2. Add remaining ingredients and stir until well combined.
3. Serve.

Nutrition: *calories 443, fat 8g, fiber1g, carbs 8g, protein 3g*

Preparation Time: 15 minutes
Cooking Time: 10 minutes
Servings: 4

109. Tabbouleh Salad

INGREDIENTS:

- 1 cup whole-wheat couscous
- 1 cup boiling water
- Zest and juice of 1 lemon
- 1 garlic clove, pressed
- Pinch sea salt
- 1 tablespoon extra-virgin olive oil, or flaxseed oil (optional)
- ½ cucumber, diced small
- 1 tomato, diced small
- 1 cup fresh parsley, chopped
- ¼ cup fresh mint, finely chopped
- 2 scallions, finely chopped
- 4 tablespoons sunflower seeds (optional)

DIRECTIONS:

1. Preparing the Ingredients.
2. Put the couscous in a medium bowl, and cover with boiling water until all the grains are submerged. Cover the bowl with a plate or wrap. Set aside.
3. Put the lemon zest and juice in a large salad bowl, then stir in the garlic, salt, and the olive oil (if using).
4. Put the cucumber, tomato, parsley, mint, and scallions in the bowl, and toss them to coat with the dressing. Take the plate off the couscous and fluff with a fork.
5. Finish and Serve
6. Add the cooked couscous to the vegetables, then toss to combine.
7. Serve topped with the sunflower seeds (if using).

Nutrition: *Calories: 304; Total fat: 11g; Carbs: 44g; Fiber: 6g; Protein: 10g*

Preparation Time: 10 minutes
Cooking Time: 30 minutes
(marinating time)
Servings: 2

110. Tuscan White Bean Salad

INGREDIENTS:

- FOR THE DRESSING
- 1 tablespoon extra-virgin olive oil
- 2 tablespoons balsamic vinegar
- 1 teaspoon minced fresh chives, or scallions
- 1 garlic clove, pressed or minced
- 1 tablespoon fresh rosemary, chopped, or 1 teaspoon dried
- 1 tablespoon fresh oregano, chopped, or 1 teaspoon dried
- Pinch sea salt
- FOR THE SALAD
- 1 (14-ounce) can cannellini beans, drained and rinsed, or 1½ cups cooked
- 6 mushrooms, thinly sliced
- 1 zucchini, diced
- 2 carrots, diced
- 2 tablespoons fresh basil, chopped

DIRECTIONS:

1. Preparing the Ingredients
2. Make the dressing by whisking all the dressing ingredients together in a large bowl.
3. Toss all the salad ingredients with the dressing.
4. Finish and Serve
5. For the best flavor, put the salad in a sealed container, shake it vigorously, then leave to marinate for 15-30 minutes.

Nutrition: *Calories: 360; Total fat: 8g; Carbs: 68g; Fiber: 15g; Protein: 18g*

Preparation Time: 30 minutes
Cooking Time: 15 minutes
Servings: 2

111. Moroccan Aubergine Salad

INGREDIENTS:

- 1 teaspoon extra-virgin olive oil
- 1 eggplant, diced
- ½ teaspoon ground cumin
- ½ teaspoon ground ginger
- ¼ teaspoon turmeric
- ¼ teaspoon ground nutmeg
- Pinch sea salt
- 1 lemon, half zested and juiced, half cut into wedges
- 2 tablespoons capers
- 1 tablespoon chopped green olives
- 1 garlic clove, pressed
- Handful fresh mint, finely chopped
- 2 cups spinach, chopped

DIRECTIONS:

1. Preparing the Ingredients
2. Heat the oil in a large skillet on medium heat, then sauté the eggplant. Once it has softened slightly, stir in the cumin, ginger, turmeric, nutmeg, and salt. Cook until the eggplant is very soft.
3. Add the lemon zest and juice, capers, olives, garlic, and mint. Sauté for another minute or two to blend the flavors. Put a handful of spinach on each plate, and spoon the eggplant mixture on top.
4. Serve with a wedge of lemon to squeeze the fresh juice over the greens.
5. To tenderize the eggplant and reduce some of its naturally occurring bitter taste, you can sweat the eggplant by salting it.
6. Finish and Serve
7. After dicing the eggplant, sprinkle it with salt and let it sit in a colander for about 30 minutes. Rinse the eggplant to remove the salt, then continue with the recipe as written.

Nutrition: *Calories: 97; Total fat: 4g; Carbs: 16g; Fiber: 8g; Protein: 4g*

Preparation Time: 10 minutes
Cooking Time: 20 minutes
Servings: 4

112. Creamy Avocado-Dressed Kale Salad

INGREDIENTS:

- FOR THE DRESSING
- 1 avocado, peeled and pitted
- 1 tablespoon fresh lemon juice, or 1 teaspoon lemon juice concentrate and 2 teaspoons water
- 1 tablespoon fresh or dried dill1 small garlic clove, pressed
- 1 scallion, chopped
- Pinch sea salt
- ¼ cup water
- FOR THE SALAD
- 8 large kale leaves
- ½ cup chopped green beans, raw or lightly steamed
- 1 cup cherry tomatoes, halved
- 1 bell pepper, chopped
- 2 scallions, chopped
- 2 cups cooked millet, or other cooked whole grain, such as quinoa or brown rice
- Hummus (optional)

DIRECTIONS:

1. TO MAKE THE DRESSING
2. Put all the ingredients in a blender or food processor. Purée until smooth, then add water as necessary to get the consistency you're looking for in your dressing. Taste for seasoning, and add more salt if you need to.
3. TO MAKE THE SALAD
4. Chop the kale, removing the stems if you want your salad less bitter, and then massage the leaves with your fingers until it wilts and gets a bit moist, about 2 minutes. You can use a pinch salt if you like to help it soften. Toss the kale with the green beans, cherry tomatoes, bell pepper, scallions, millet, and

Nutrition: *Calories: 225; Total fat: 7g; Carbs: 37g; Fiber: 7g; Protein: 7g*

Preparation Time: 10 minutes
Cooking Time: 0 minutes
Servings: 4

113. Spinach and Avocado Salad

INGREDIENTS:

- 2 spring onions, chopped
- 2 avocados, peeled, pitted and cubed
- 3 plum tomatoes, chopped
- 10 ounces spinach, chopped
- A pinch of black pepper
- A pinch of salt
- 1 tablespoon olive oil
- 1 tablespoon chives
- Juice of 1 lime

DIRECTIONS:

1. In a bowl, mix the spinach with tomatoes and the other ingredients, toss and serve.

Nutrition: *calories 185, fat 4, fiber 5.4, carbs 6.4, protein 7*

Preparation Time: 15 minutes
Cooking Time: 30 minutes
Servings: 4

114. Cobb Salad

INGREDIENTS:

- 8 romaine lettuce leaves (chopped)
- 1 avocado
- 1 ½ cups of cherry tomatoes (chopped)
- 1 cup of corn
- ½ cup of hummus (plain)
- 1 block of tofu (350g and firm)
- 3 tbsp of olive oil
- 2 ½ tbsp of dill (chopped)
- 2 tbsp of nutritional yeast
- 2 tbsp of low-sodium soy sauce
- 1 ¼ tsp of agave nectar
- ½ cup of mushrooms (chopped)

DIRECTIONS:

1. Set the oven to 375 F and prepare 2 baking sheets with a single layer of parchment paper. Mix nutritional yeast, 1 tbsp soy sauce, and 1 tbsp olive oil in a bowl.
2. Break the tofu into cube-sized chunks, and add it to the ingredients in the bowl. Mix the ingredients.
3. Place the tofu evenly on the baking sheets, and bake it for 25 to 30 minutes while turning it over every 10 minutes.
4. While the tofu bakes in the oven, mix the 2 tbsp of olive oil, 2 tbsp of soy sauce, and the agave nectar in a bowl. Add the mushrooms to the bowl, and combine the ingredients.
5. Add the marinated mushrooms to the tofu in the oven, and bake it for 20 minutes.
6. Plate the romaine lettuce in a large bowl, and top it with the mushrooms, cherry tomatoes, tofu, corn, and avocado. Assemble the salad ingredients neatly to make it look extra delicious.

Nutrition: *Calories: 270, Carbohydrates: 21g, Protein: 8g, Fat: 19g*

Preparation Time: 5 minutes
Cooking Time: 5 minutes
Servings: 4

115. Caesar Salad

INGREDIENTS:

- 4 romaine lettuce hearts (large)
- 2 Seitan tenders: ½ cup of vital wheat gluten, 1 ¼ tbsp of water, 1 ¼ tbsp of nutritional yeast, 200g of tofu (soft), ¾ tbsp of onion powder, 1 ¼ tsp of vegetable broth powder, ¾ tsp of garlic powder, ¼ tsp of salt
- 2 cups of croutons (vegan)
- 1 tbsp of sesame oil
- 2 tbsp of parmesan (vegan)
- Seasoning:
- ½ cup of cashews
- ½ cup of water
- 2 tbsp of nutritional yeast
- ¼ cup of lemon juice
- 1 tbsp of Dijon mustard
- 1 garlic clove

Nutrition: *Calories: 300, Carbohydrates: 24g, Protein: 20g, Fat: 15g*

DIRECTIONS:

1. To make the vegan seitan tenders, add the vital wheat gluten, water, nutritional yeast, tofu, onion powder, vegetable broth powder, garlic powder, and salt to a food processor and put it on high speed until it forms a ball of dough.
2. Dust a working surface, like an extra-large chopping board or counter surface with vital wheat gluten. Place the bowl in the wheat, and dust the top of the dough until it becomes soft.
3. Cut the dough into 4 pieces, and using your fingers, press every piece into an oval shape.
4. Add water to a pot, about ¼ full, with a steamer basket on top at medium-high heat. Allow the water to simmer and grease the basket with some olive oil.
5. Spray the tenders out onto the basket, and cover them. Cook for 25 minutes. Flip it halfway to cook on the other side. Cover the cooked seitan, and place it in an airtight container, allowing it to chill for 1 hour.
6. While the seitan tenders are chilling in the refrigerator, make the seasoning by soaking the cashews in water for 10 minutes, draining, and rinsing it before blending all of the ingredients at high speed.
7. Remove the seitan tenders from the refrigerator after 1 hour, and marinate them in the seasoning. Add the seitan tenders to a pan with sesame oil over medium-high heat. Allow it to fry within a few minutes on both sides, and then slice it into strips.
8. Shred the romaine lettuce and add to a large salad bowl. Add the tender seitan strips to it with croutons, vegan parmesan, and the remaining salad dressing.
9. Serve the salad fresh or store it in 4 separate mason jars or sealed containers for 3 days.

Preparation Time: 15 minutes
Cooking Time: 60 minutes (chill time)
Servings: 6

116. Basil Mango Jicama Salad

INGREDIENTS:

- 1 jicama, peeled and grated
- 1 mango, peeled and sliced
- ¼ cup non-dairy milk
- 2 tablespoons fresh basil, chopped
- 1 large scallion, chopped
- ⅛ teaspoon sea salt
- 1½ tablespoons tahini (optional)
- Fresh greens (for serving)
- Chopped cashews (optional, for serving)
- Cheesy Sprinkle (optional, for serving)

DIRECTIONS:

1. Preparing the Ingredients
2. Put the jicama in a large bowl.
3. Purée the mango in a food processor or blender, with just enough non-dairy milk to make a thick sauce.
4. Add the basil, scallions, and salt. Stir in the tahini if you want to make a thicker, creamier, and more filling sauce.
5. Pour the dressing over the jicama and marinate, covered in the fridge for 1 hour or more to break down some of the starch.
6. Finish and Serve
7. Serve over a bed of greens, topped with chopped cashews and/or cheesy sprinkle (if using).

Nutrition: *Calories: 76; Total fat: 2g; Carbs: 14g; Fiber: 5g; Protein: 1g*

Preparation Time: 5 minutes
Cooking Time: 0 minutes
Servings: 1

117. Apple-Sunflower Spinach Salad

INGREDIENTS:

- 1 cup baby spinach
- ½ apple, cored and chopped
- ¼ red onion, thinly sliced (optional)
- 2 tablespoons sunflower seeds or Cinnamon-Lime Sunflower Seeds
- 2 tablespoons dried cranberries
- 2 tablespoons Raspberry Vinaigrette

DIRECTIONS:

1. Preparing the Ingredients.
2. Arrange the spinach on a plate. Top with the apple, red onion (if using), sunflower seeds, and cranberries, and drizzle with the vinaigrette.

Nutrition: *Calories: 444; Protein: 7g; Total fat: 28g; Saturated fat: 3g; Carbohydrates: 53g; Fiber: 8g*

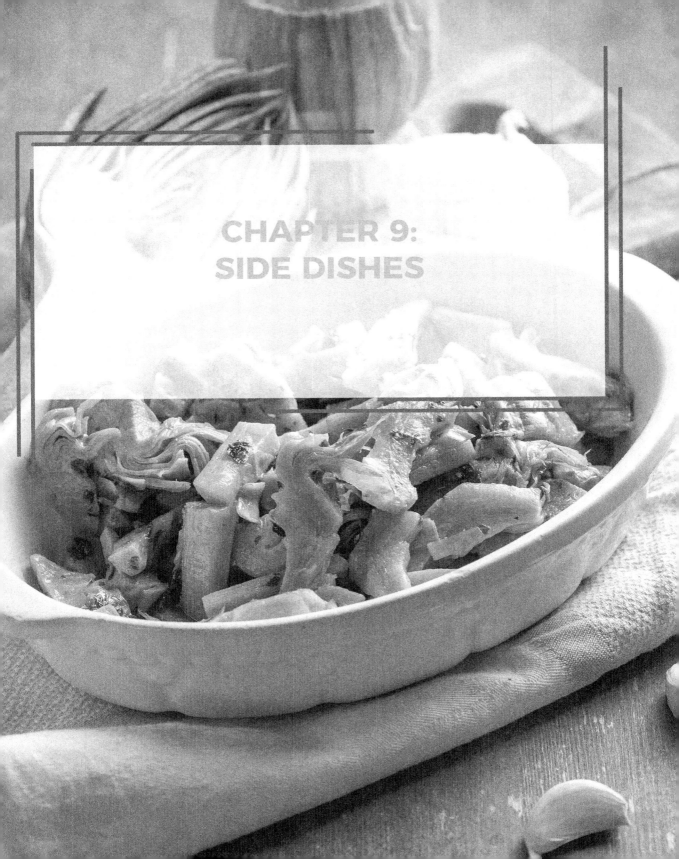

CHAPTER 9:
SIDE DISHES

Preparation Time: 10 minutes
Cooking Time: 00 minutes
Servings: 4

118. Balsamic Beans Salad

INGREDIENTS:

- 1 cup of frozen green beans
- 1/4 cup chopped almonds
- 1/2 cup chopped green onions
- 3/4 cup mayonnaise
- 2 tablespoons balsamic vinegar
- Black pepper to taste

DIRECTIONS:

1. Place beans in a colander, and run warm water over them until they are thawed. Place in a large bowl.
2. Toast almonds in a skillet over medium heat. Then combine with beans.
3. Stir in onions, and mayonnaise. Mix in balsamic vinegar, and season with pepper. Cover, and refrigerator.

Nutrition: *Calories: 145; Total Fat: 10.9g; Saturated Fat: 2.6g; Cholesterol: 14mg; Sodium: 263mg; Total Carbohydrate: 9.4g; Dietary Fiber: 1.5g; Total Sugars: 3.1g; Protein: 3.3g; Calcium: 67mg; Iron: 1mg; Potassium: 94mg; Phosphorus: 44mg*

Preparation Time: 10 minutes
Cooking Time: 50 minutes
Servings: 4

119. Farro Side Dish

INGREDIENTS:

- 1 tsp. lemon juice
- A pinch salt and black pepper
- 1 cup cherries, pitted
- 10 mint leaves, chopped
- 1 tbsp. balsamic vinegar
- 1 cup farro
- 3 cups water
- 1 tbsp. olive oil
- 1/4 cup chives, chopped

DIRECTION

1. Put farro and water in your instant pot. Cover and cook on High for 40 minutes.
2. Drain the farro and transfer to a bowl.
3. Add vinegar, oil, lemon juice, salt, pepper, cherries, mint and chives.
4. Toss well and divide amongst plates. Serve and enjoy!

Nutrition: *Calories 393 kcal Fats 17. 1g Carbs 31. 9g Protein 27. 8g*

Preparation Time: 10 minutes
Cooking Time: 13 minutes
Servings: 4

120. Flavored Polenta

INGREDIENTS:

- 1/3 cup sun-dried tomatoes, chopped
- 2 tbsp. olive oil
- 1/2 cup onion, chopped
- 2 tsp. oregano, chopped
- 1 tsp. rosemary, chopped
- 1 cup polenta
- 1 bay leaf
- A pinch salt
- 4 cups veggie stock
- 2 tsp. garlic, minced
- 2 tbsp. parsley, chopped
- 3 tbsp. basil, chopped

DIRECTION

1. Set your instant pot on sauté mode. Add oil and heat it up.
2. Add onion, stir and cook for 1 minute.
3. Add garlic, stir and cook for 1 minute more.
4. Add sun-dried tomatoes, stock, salt, bay leaf, rosemary, oregano, half of the parsley, half of the basil and the polenta.
5. Stir, cover and cook on High for 5 minutes.
6. Discard bay leaf, stir polenta, add the rest of the basil and parsley.
7. Leave everything aside for a few minutes more.
8. Divide amongst plates and serve. Enjoy!

Nutrition: *calories 221, fat 11.9, fiber 2.5, carbs 10.4, protein 22.6*

Preparation Time: 10 minutes
Cooking Time: 30 minutes
Servings: 4

121. Fried Cabbage

INGREDIENTS:

- 1 cabbage head, sliced
- 1 yellow onion, chopped
- 2 tsps. stevia
- 2 tsps. balsamic vinegar
- 3 garlic cloves, minced
- 1 tbsp. olive oil
- A pinch of salt and black pepper
- 2 tsps. mustard

DIRECTIONS:

1. Heat oil on Sauté. Add onion and garlic and cook for 2 minutes. Add cabbage, stevia, vinegar, mustard, salt, and pepper. Mix and cover. Cook on High for 4 minutes. Stir and serve.

Nutrition: *calories 221, fat 11.9, fiber 2.5, carbs 10.4, protein 22.6*

Preparation Time: **10 minutes**
Cooking Time: **20 minutes**
Servings: **4**

122. Garlic Artichokes

INGREDIENTS:

- 4 artichokes, trimmed and stems removed
- 4 tsp. olive oil
- 1/2 cup veggie stock
- 2 tsp. garlic, minced
- A pinch salt

DIRECTION

1. Put the artichokes in your instant pot. Add garlic, a pinch of salt and oil. Toss them a bit.
2. Add the stock, cover the pot and cook on High for 7 minutes.
3. Divide amongst plates. Serve and enjoy!

Nutrition: *Calories: 150 Cal Fat: 4 g Carbs: 21 g Protein: 10 g Fiber: 2 g*

Preparation Time: **10 minutes**
Cooking Time: **30 minutes**
Servings: **4**

123. Green Beans Side Dish

INGREDIENTS:

- 1-pound green beans, trimmed
- 8 ounces white mushrooms, sliced
- 1 yellow onion, chopped
- 2 tbsps. olive oil
- ½ cup veggie stock
- 2 tbsps. flax meal
- A pinch of salt and black pepper

DIRECTIONS:

1. Heat oil in the Instant Pot on Sauté. Add onion and cook for 1 minute. Add half of the stock and mushrooms. Mix and cook for 1 minute. Add rest of the stock, green beans, salt, pepper, and flax meal. Mix and cover. Cook on High for 2 minutes. Serve.

Nutrition: *Calories: 150 Cal Fat: 4 g Carbs: 21 g Protein: 10 g Fiber: 2 g*

Preparation Time: 10 minutes
Cooking Time: 90 minutes
Servings: 4

124. Instant Pot Peanuts

INGREDIENTS:

- 3 garlic cloves
- 1 tbsp. palm sugar
- 1 pound raw peanuts, rinsed well
- 3 cinnamon sticks
- 3 tbsp. salt
- 3 star anise
- 4 red hot chili peppers

DIRECTION

1. Put peanuts in your instant pot. Add water to cover, cinnamon stick, salt, anise, sugar and chili pepper.
2. Stir, cover and cook on High for 1 hour and 20 minutes.
3. Release pressure naturally. Leave aside for 20 minutes.
4. Transfer the peanuts to a serving bowl. Serve and enjoy!

Nutrition: *Calories 393 kcal Fats 17. 1g Carbs 31. 9g Protein 27. 8g*

Preparation Time: 10 minutes
Cooking Time: 30 minutes
Servings: 4

125. Italian Appetizer Salad

INGREDIENTS:

- 10 cherry tomatoes, halved
- 2 tbsp. pine nuts
- 1/4 cup olive oil
- 1 eggplant, cubed
- A pinch salt and black pepper
- 1 yellow onion, cut into medium pieces
- 1 red bell pepper, chopped
- 2 potatoes, cubed
- 2 zucchinis, cut into rounds
- 1 tbsp. capers
- 1/4 cup black olives, pitted and sliced
- 1 tbsp. raisins
- 1 bunch basil, chopped

DIRECTION

1. Set your instant pot on Sauté mode. Add oil and heat it up.
2. Add eggplant and onion. Stir and cook for 2 minutes.
3. Add bell pepper, potatoes, zucchinis, a pinch of salt and black pepper.
4. Stir and cook for 2 minutes more.
5. Add capers, tomatoes, olives, raisins and 1 tablespoon pine nuts.
6. Stir, cover and cook on High for 4 minutes.
7. Add basil and the rest of the pine nuts.
8. Toss and divide into plates. Serve and enjoy!

Nutrition: *Calories: 150 Cal Fat: 4 g Carbs: 21 g Protein: 10 g Fiber: 2 g*

Preparation Time: **7 minutes**
Cooking Time: **8 minutes**
Servings: **4**

126. Lemon Potatoes

INGREDIENTS:

- 4 white potatoes
- 1 teaspoon lemon zest
- 1 teaspoon Pink salt
- 1 tablespoon fresh dill, chopped
- 1 teaspoon dried oregano
- 2 tablespoon lemon juice
- ¼ cup vegetable broth
- 1 tablespoon olive oil

DIRECTIONS:

1. Wash potatoes carefully and chop roughly.
2. Whisk together lemon juice, olive oil, dried oregano, and fresh dill.
3. Pour olive oil mixture over the potatoes and sprinkle with salt. Shake well and transfer in the instant pot.
4. Add vegetable broth and cook on Manual mode for 8 minutes.
5. Allow natural pressure release.

Nutrition: *calories 185, fat 3.9, fiber 5.4, carbs 34.5, protein 4.2*

Preparation Time: **10 minutes**
Cooking Time: **30 minutes**
Servings: **4**

127. Lentil Party Mix

INGREDIENTS:

- A pinch salt and black pepper
- 2 tsp. mustard powder
- 2 tsp. garlic powder
- 2 carrots, chopped
- 1 cup water
- 1/4 cup apple cider vinegar
- 1/2 cup maple syrup
- 1 tsp. chili powder
- 2 cups lentils
- 1 yellow onion, chopped
- 4 cups tomato puree
- 2 tsp. cumin, ground

DIRECTION

1. In your instant pot, mix carrots with water, lentils, onion, tomato puree, vinegar, maple syrup, chili powder, salt, pepper, mustard powder, garlic powder and cumin.
2. Stir, cover and cook on High for 20 minutes.
3. Divide into small bowls. Serve and enjoy!

Nutrition: *Calories 393 kcal Fats 17. 1g Carbs 31. 9g Protein 27. 8g*

Preparation Time: 10 minutes
Cooking Time: 30 minutes
Servings: 4

128. Mashed Cauliflower and Chives

INGREDIENTS:

- 2 tsp. olive oil
- A pinch salt and black pepper
- 1/2 tsp. turmeric powder
- 1 1/2 cups water
- 1 1/2 cups water
- 1 cauliflower head, florets separated
- 3 chives, chopped

DIRECTION

1. Put the water in your instant pot. Add steamer basket and then put the cauliflower inside.
2. Cover and cook on High for 6 minutes.
3. Transfer cauliflower to a bowl. Mash with a potato masher and transfer to your food processor.
4. Add salt, pepper, chives, turmeric and oil. Blend well.
5. Divide amongst serving plates. Serve and enjoy!

Nutrition: *Calories: 150 Cal Fat: 4 g Carbs: 21 g Protein: 10 g Fiber: 2 g*

Preparation Time: 5 minutes
Cooking Time: 4 minutes
Servings: 4

129. Mongolian Stir Fry

INGREDIENTS:

- 1 tablespoon minced ginger
- 1 teaspoon minced garlic
- 1 tablespoon avocado oil
- 4 tablespoons soy sauce
- 1 teaspoon chili flakes
- 1 teaspoon cornstarch
- 1 tablespoon brown sugar
- 8 tablespoon water
- ½ teaspoon cayenne pepper
- 1-pound seitan, chopped

DIRECTIONS:

1. In the mixing bowl whisk together minced ginger, minced garlic, avocado oil, soy sauce, chili flakes, cornstarch, brown sugar, cayenne pepper, and water.
2. Preheat instant pot bowl on Saute mode until hot.
3. Transfer ginger mixture in the instant pot and cook it for 1 minute.
4. Then add chopped seitan and stir well.
5. Close the lid and set Manual mode (high pressure) for 1 minute. Use quick pressure release.
6. Mix up the side dish well before serving.

Nutrition: *calories 59, fat 0.9, fiber 0.8, carbs 5.6, protein 6.6*

Preparation Time: 10 minutes
Cooking Time: 30 minutes
Servings: 4

130. Mushroom Rice Pilaf

INGREDIENTS:

- ¼ cup butter
- 1 cup medium-grain rice
- ½ lb. sliced baby portobello mushrooms
- 6 green onions, chopped
- 2 garlic cloves, minced
- 1 cup of water
- 4 tsps. better than bouillon vegetarian

DIRECTIONS:

1. Melt the butter on Sauté in the Instant Pot. Add rice and cook for 5 minutes. Add garlic, green onions, and mushrooms.
2. In a bowl, whisk the water and bouillon. Pour over rice mixture.
3. Cover and cook on High for 4 minutes. Open and serve

Nutrition: *Calories: 150 Cal Fat: 4 g Carbs: 21 g Protein: 10 g Fiber: 2 g*

Preparation Time: 10 minutes
Cooking Time: 30 minutes
Servings: 4

131. Mustard Glazed Carrots

INGREDIENTS:

- 1/4 tsp. baking soda
- 1 tsp. thyme, dried
- 1 tbsp. mustard
- 1 tbsp. olive oil
- 3 pounds carrots, cut into medium strips
- 1 tbsp. maple syrup
- 2 tbsp. veggie stock

DIRECTION

1. Set your instant pot on Sauté mode. Add oil and heat up.
2. Add maple syrup, mustard, baking soda and veggie stock.
3. Stir and cook for 1 minute.
4. Add carrots and thyme. Stir a bit.
5. Cover and cook on High for 4 minutes.
6. Divide amongst plates. Serve and enjoy!

Nutrition: *Calories: 150 Cal Fat: 4 g Carbs: 21 g Protein: 10 g Fiber: 2 g*

Preparation Time: 10 minutes
Cooking Time: 30 minutes
Servings: 4

132. Onions Appetizer

INGREDIENTS:

- 1 tbsp. flaxseed mixed well with 2 tbsp. water
- 3 tbsp. thyme, finely chopped
- Salt and pepper, to taste
- 12 small red onions
- 2 cups veggie stock
- 5 potatoes, peeled and chopped
- 4 cups water
- 3/4 cup vegan cheese, grated

DIRECTION

1. Put potatoes in your instant pot. Add half of the water and cook on High for 15 minutes.
2. Cut the top of each onion, cut a base and scoop out some of the insides.
3. Release the pressure naturally from pot.
4. Drain potatoes, transfer them to a bowl and mash them.
5. Add flaxseed, salt, pepper and thyme and stir everything.
6. Fill the onions with potatoes mix and arrange them in the steamer basket of your instant pot.
7. Add the rest of the water and the stock on the bottom.
8. Sprinkle vegan cheese, cover and cook on High for 10 more minutes.
9. Release pressure naturally.
10. Arrange onions on a platter and serve warm. Enjoy!

Nutrition: *Calories: 150 Cal Fat: 4 g Carbs: 21 g Protein: 10 g Fiber: 2 g*

Preparation Time: 10 minutes
Cooking Time: 30 minutes
Servings: 4

133. Pearl Onion Appetizer

INGREDIENTS:

- 1/2 cup water
- 1 bay leaf
- 1 pound pearl onions, peeled
- A pinch salt and black pepper
- 4 tbsp. balsamic vinegar
- 1 tbsp. coconut flour
- 1 tbsp. stevia

DIRECTION

1. In your instant pot, mix pearl onions with salt, pepper, water and bay leaf.
2. Cover and cook on Low for 5 minutes. Meanwhile, heat up a pan over medium heat.
3. Add vinegar, stevia and flour, stir, bring to a simmer and take off heat.
4. Pour this over pearl onions.
5. Toss and divide into bowls. Serve and enjoy!

Nutrition: *calories 304, fat 10.3, fiber 5.4, carbs 46.8, protein 8.4*

Preparation Time: 10 minutes
Cooking Time: 30 minutes

134. Pickled Green Peppers

INGREDIENTS:

- 1 1/2 tsp. stevia
- 1 1/2 cups apple cider vinegar
- 1 tsp. pickling salt
- 1 pound green chilies, sliced
- 1/4 tsp. garlic powder

DIRECTION

1. Put green chilies in your instant pot.
2. Add pickling salt, stevia, vinegar and garlic powder.
3. Stir, cover and cook on High for 1 minute.
4. Divide into jars and serve cold. Enjoy!

Nutrition: *calories 304, fat 10.3, fiber 5.4, carbs 46.8, protein 8.4*

Preparation Time: 5 minutes
Cooking Time: 8 minutes
Servings: 4

135. Pineapple Rice

INGREDIENTS:

- 1 ½ cup of rice
- 2 cups of water
- 1 cup pineapple juice
- 1 can pineapples, chopped
- 1 teaspoon coconut cream

DIRECTIONS:

1. Pour water and pineapple juice in the instant pot. Add rice and chopped pineapple, and close the lid.
2. Set Manual mode (high pressure) for 8 minutes. Then use quick pressure release.
3. Transfer the cooked pineapple rice in the bowl and add coconut cream. Stir it.

Nutrition: *calories 310, fat 0.9, fiber 1.6, carbs 69, protein 5.4*

Preparation Time: 10 minutes
Cooking Time: 30 minutes
Servings: 4

136. Quinoa Side Dish

INGREDIENTS:

- 2 cups quinoa
- 3 cups of water
- Juice of 1 lemon
- A pinch of salt and black pepper
- A handful of mixed parsley, cilantro, and basil, chopped

DIRECTIONS:

1. In the pot, mix quinoa with water, lemon, salt, pepper, and mixed herbs. Stir and cover. Cook on High for 2 minutes. Leave quinoa aside for 10 minutes. Fluff and serve

Nutritions *Calories 109, Cal Fat 2 g, Carbs 13 g, Protein 1 g, Fiber 0 g*

Preparation Time: 15 minutes
Cooking Time: 3 minutes
Servings: .3

137. Quinoa with Basil and Lemongrass

INGREDIENTS:

- 1 cup quinoa
- 1 cup vegetable broth
- 1 tablespoon lemongrass, chopped
- 1 teaspoon dried basil
- 1 tablespoon almond butter
- ¾ teaspoon ground nutmeg
- 1/3 teaspoon Pink salt

DIRECTIONS:

1. Put quinoa in an instant pot.
2. Add vegetable broth, ground nutmeg, and salt. Close the lid, seal it, and set Manual mode (high pressure).
3. Cook quinoa for 3 minutes and allow natural pressure release for 10 minutes.
4. In the cooked quinoa add almond butter, lemongrass and dried basil. Mix the side dish up.
5. The side dish is cooked.

Nutrition: *calories 259, fat 7.1, fiber 4.6, carbs 38.4, protein 10.8*

138. Ratatouille

INGREDIENTS:

- 1 cup tomatoes, chopped
- 3 sweet peppers, chopped
- 1 red onion, diced
- 2 garlic cloves, peeled
- 1 zucchini, chopped
- ½ eggplant, chopped
- 2 tablespoons sesame oil
- 1 tablespoon fresh parsley, chopped
- 1 teaspoon tomato paste
- 1 teaspoon dried cilantro
- ¼ teaspoon dried oregano
- 1 tablespoon Italian seasoning
- 1 jalapeno, pepper, chopped
- 2 cups vegetable broth

DIRECTIONS:

1. Set instant pot on Saute mode for 8 minutes and pour sesame oil.
2. Add sweet peppers, tomatoes, and onions. Stir the mixture.
3. Then add zucchini, garlic clove, eggplant, and jalapeno pepper.
4. Mix up the vegetables and keep cooking.
5. Add parsley, dried oregano, Italian seasoning, and tomato paste.
6. When the time of sauteing is over – add vegetable broth and close the lid.
7. Cook the meal on Manual mode (High pressure) for 2 minutes. Allow natural pressure release for 5 minutes.

Nutrition: *calories 110, fat 6.1, fiber 3.4, carbs 12, protein 3.6*

139. Red Cabbage with Apples

INGREDIENTS:

- 1-pound red cabbage
- 1 apple, chopped
- 1 teaspoon salt
- ¼ cup of coconut milk
- ¾ cup almond milk
- ½ teaspoon chili flakes

DIRECTIONS:

1. Shred red cabbage and mix it up with salt.
2. Transfer the mixture in the instant pot. Add coconut milk, almond milk, and chili flakes.
3. Then add apple and set manual mode (High pressure).
4. Cook the cabbage for 7 minutes. Then allow natural pressure release.
5. Transfer the meal into the serving bowls and mix up well before serving.

Nutrition: *calories 123, fat 5.1, fiber 6, carbs 20.2, protein 2.6*

140. Roasted Potatoes

INGREDIENTS:

- 1/2 tsp. onion powder
- 1/4 tsp. sweet paprika
- 1 1/2 pounds potatoes, cut into wedges
- 1/4 cup avocado oil
- A pinch salt and black pepper
- 1 cup veggie stock
- 1 tsp. garlic powder

DIRECTION

1. Add the oil to your instant pot. Set it to Sauté mode and heat the oil up.
2. Add potatoes and cook them for 8 minutes.
3. Add salt, pepper, onion powder, garlic powder, paprika and stock.
4. Toss a bit, cover pot and cook on High for 7 minutes.
5. Divide potatoes amongst plates. Serve and enjoy!

Nutrition: *Calories 393 kcal Fats 17. 1g Carbs 31. 9g Protein 27. 8g*

141. Rosemary Beets

INGREDIENTS:

- 5 large fresh beets, scrubbed and trimmed
- 1 tbsp. olive oil
- 1 medium red onion, chopped
- 2 garlic cloves, minced
- 1 medium orange, peeled and chopped
- 1/3 cup honey
- 1/4 cup white balsamic vinegar
- 1 tbsp. minced fresh rosemary
- 2 tsps. minced fresh thyme
- 3/4 tsp. salt
- 1/2 tsp. Chinese five-spice powder
- 1/2 tsp. coarsely ground pepper
- 1 cup crumbled feta cheese
- 1 cup water for the pot

DIRECTIONS:

1. Place the trivet and 1 cup water in the pot. Place the beets on the trivet and cover. Cook on High for 20 minutes.
2. Open and remove beets. Clean the pot. Peel and cut beets into wedges. Heat the oil on Sauté. Cook onions for 5 minutes. Add garlic and cook for 1 minute more.
3. Stir in honey, orange, vinegar, rosemary, thyme, salt, spice, pepper, and beets. Heat through and sprinkle with cheese. Serve.

Nutrition: *Calories 393 kcal Fats 17. 1g Carbs 31. 9g Protein 27. 8g*

Preparation Time: 10 minutes
Cooking Time: 30 minutes

142. Simple Roasted Potatoes

INGREDIENTS:

- 1 and ½ pounds potatoes, cut into wedges
- ¼ cup avocado oil
- A pinch of salt and black pepper
- ½ tsp. onion powder
- ¼ tsp. sweet paprika
- 1 cup veggie stock
- 1 tsp. garlic powder

DIRECTIONS:

1. Heat oil on Sauté. Add potatoes and cook for 8 minutes. Add the remaining ingredients and mix. Cover and cook on High for 7 minutes. Serve.

Nutrition: *calories 304, fat 10.3, fiber 5.4, carbs 46.8, protein 8.4*

Preparation Time: 10 minutes
Cooking Time: 3 minutes
Servings: 4

143. Spaghetti Squash with Tomatoes

INGREDIENTS:

- 1 medium spaghetti squash, halved lengthwise, seeds removed
- 1 can (14 oz.) diced tomatoes, drained
- ¼ cup sliced green olives with pimientos
- 1 tsp. dried oregano
- ½ tsp. salt
- ½ tsp. pepper
- ½ cup shredded cheddar cheese
- ¼ cup minced fresh basil
- 1 cup water for the pot

DIRECTIONS:

1. Place a trivet in the pot and add 1 cup of water. Place squash on the trivet. Cover and cook on High for 7 minutes.
2. Do a quick release and open. Remove squash and clean the pot. Use a fork to make spaghetti from the squash. Discard skin.
3. Return squash to the pot. Add tomatoes, olives, oregano, salt, and pepper.
4. Cook on Sauté for 3 minutes. Top with cheese and basil and serve.

Nutrition: *Calories 393 kcal Fats 17. 1g Carbs 31. 9g Protein 27. 8g*

Preparation Time: 10 minutes
Cooking Time: 5 minutes
Servings: 4

144. Steamed Leeks

INGREDIENTS:

- 1 large tomato, chopped
- 1 small navel orange, chopped
- 2 tbsps. minced fresh parsley
- 2 tbsps. sliced olives
- 1 tsp. capers, drained
- 1 tsp. red wine vinegar
- 1 tsp. olive oil
- ½ tsp. grated orange zest
- ½ tsp. pepper
- 6 medium leeks (white portion only), halved lengthwise, cleaned
- Crumbled feta cheese for serving
- 1 cup water for the pot

DIRECTIONS:

1. Combine the first 9 ingredients.
2. Set aside. Place a trivet in the pot and add 1 cup of water. Place leeks on the trivet and close the pot.
3. Cook on High for 2 minutes. Do a quick release and open.
4. Transfer leeks to a platter. Spoon tomato mixture on top. Sprinkle with cheese and serve.

Nutrition: *Calories 393 kcal Fats 17. 1g Carbs 31. 9g Protein 27. 8g*

Preparation Time: 10 minutes
Cooking Time: 2 minutes
Servings: 4

145. Summer Squash, and Zucchini with Cheese

INGREDIENTS:

- 1 lb. medium yellow summer squash, chopped
- 1 lb. medium zucchini, chopped
- 2 medium tomatoes, chopped
- 1 cup vegetable broth
- ¼ cup thinly sliced green onions
- ½ tsp. salt
- ¼ tsp. pepper
- 1 ½ cups Caesar salad croutons, coarsely crushed
- ½ cup shredded cheddar cheese

DIRECTIONS:

1. Place the squash, tomatoes, broth, green onions, salt, and pepper to the Instant Pot. Cover and cook on High for 2 minutes.
2. Open and serve topped with croutons, and cheese.

Nutrition: *calories 304, fat 10.3, fiber 5.4, carbs 46.8, protein 8.4*

Preparation Time: 10 minutes
Cooking Time: 30 minutes
Servings: 4

146. Sweet Brussels Sprouts

INGREDIENTS:

- 2 pounds Brussels sprouts, trimmed
- 1 tbsp. olive oil
- 1 tsp. orange zest, grated
- ¼ cup orange juice
- 2 tbsps. stevia
- A pinch of salt and black pepper

DIRECTIONS:

1. Heat oil in the pot on Sauté. Add sprouts and cook for 1 minute. Add orange zest, juice, stevia, salt, and pepper. Mix and cover. Cook on High for 4 minutes. Open and serve

Nutrion *Calories: 109 Cal Fat: 2 g Carbs: 13 g Protein: 1 g Fiber: 0 g*

Preparation Time: 10 minutes
Cooking Time: 5 minutes
Servings: 4

147. Red Cabbage Salad

INGREDIENTS:

- 2 cups red cabbage, shredded
- 1 tbsp. olive oil
- Salt and black pepper to the taste
- ¼ cup white onion, finely chopped
- 2 tsps. red wine vinegar
- ½ teaspoon sugar
- Water as needed

DIRECTIONS:

1. Put cabbage in the pot and add water. Cover and cook on High for 5 minutes. Open and drain water.
2. Transfer cabbage to a bowl. Add salt, pepper, onion, oil, sugar, and vinegar. Mix and serve.

Nutrition: *Calories 150; Carbs 12g; Fat 2g; Protein 3g*

148. Brussels Sprouts Salad

Preparation Time: 10 minutes
Cooking Time: 30 minutes
Servings: 4

INGREDIENTS:

- 1-pound Brussels sprouts, trimmed and halved
- ¼ cup cashew nuts, chopped
- ½ tbsp. unsalted butter, melted
- ¼ cup almonds, chopped
- 1 cup pomegranate seeds
- 1 cup of water
- Salt and black pepper, to taste

DIRECTIONS:

1. Place the trivet in the pot and add water. Season Brussels sprout with salt and pepper and place on the trivet. Cook on High for 4 minutes.
2. Open and top with melted butter, almonds, cashew nuts, and pomegranate seeds. Mix and serve

Nutrition: *Calories 170; Carbs 20.4g; Fat 8.8g; Protein 6.7g*

149. Chickpea Greek Salad

Preparation Time: 10 minutes
Cooking Time: 30 minutes
Servings: 4

INGREDIENTS:

- 1 cup of dried chickpeas, soaked overnight, then drained
- 3 cups of water
- 2 tbsps. extra-virgin olive oil
- 1 tbsp. red wine vinegar
- 1 tsp. kosher salt
- ½ tsp. ground black pepper
- ½ cup of finely minced onion
- 10 cherry tomatoes, cut in half
- 10 pitted black olives, cut in half
- 1 cucumber, cut into ½ -inch dice
- ¼ cup of chopped green bell pepper
- 2 tbsp. finely minced cilantro
- 1 ounce of crumbled feta cheese

DIRECTIONS:

1. Pour the water into the pot and add the chickpeas. Cover and cook on High for 15 minutes. Open and drain.
2. Cool. In a bowl, combine the oil, vinegar, salt, and black pepper. Mix well. In another bowl, combine the chickpeas, onion, tomatoes, olives, cucumber, bell pepper, and cilantro. Mix and top with feta. Serve

Nutrition: *Calories 107; Carbs 8g; Fat 7g; Protein 3g*

Preparation Time: 10 minutes
Cooking Time: 30 minutes
Servings: 4

150. Beans and Greens Salad

INGREDIENTS:

- ¾ cup toasted pistachios
- 6 cups of arugula
- 3 tbsps. olive oil
- 2 tbsps. lemon juice
- 1 (15.5-ounce) can cannellini beans
- Salt and black pepper, to taste

DIRECTIONS:

1. Place the beans, salt, and pepper in the pot and cover. Cook on High for 20 minutes. Open. In a bowl, mix the lemon juice, oil, salt, and pepper. Add beans, pistachios, and arugula. Serve.

Nutrition: *Calories 267; Carbs 29g; Fat 11g; Protein 13g*

Preparation Time: 10 minutes
Cooking Time: 00 minutes
Servings: 4

151. Kale and Cauliflower Salad

INGREDIENTS:

- ½ cup lemon juice
- 1 tablespoon olive oil
- 1 teaspoon honey
- 1/8 teaspoon salt
- ¼ teaspoon ground black pepper
- 1 bunch kale, cut into bite-size pieces
- ½ cup roasted cauliflower
- ½ cup dried cranberries

DIRECTIONS:

1. Whisk lemon juice, olive oil, honey, salt, and black pepper in a large bowl. Add kale, cauliflower, and cranberries; toss to combine.

Nutrition: *Calories: 76; Total Fat: 5g; Saturated Fat: 1.2g; Cholesterol: 2mg; Sodium: 131mg; Total Carbohydrate: 5.9g; Dietary Fiber: 1.3g; Total Sugars: 2.8g; Protein: 1.8g; Calcium: 59mg; Iron: 1mg; Potassium: 146mg; Phosphorus: 88mg*

Preparation Time: 10 minutes
Cooking Time: 25 minutes
Servings: 4

152. Black Bean Meatball Salad

INGREDIENTS:

- For the Meatballs:
- 1/2 cup quinoa, cooked
- 1 cup cooked black beans
- 3 cloves of garlic, peeled
- 1 small red onion, peeled
- 1 teaspoon ground dried coriander
- 1 teaspoon ground dried cumin
- 1 teaspoon smoked paprika
- For the Salad:
- 1 large sweet potato, peeled, diced
- 1 lemon, juiced
- 1 teaspoon minced garlic
- 1 cup coriander leaves
- 1/3 cup almonds
- 1/3 teaspoon ground black pepper
- ½ teaspoon salt
- 1 1/2 tablespoons olive oil

Nutrition: *Calories: 140 Cal; Fat: 8 g; Carbs: 8 g; Protein: 10 g; Fiber: 4 g*

DIRECTIONS:

1. Prepare the meatballs and for this, place beans and puree in a blender, pulse until pureed, and place this mixture in a medium bowl.
2. Add onion and garlic, process until chopped, add to the bean mixture, add all the spices, stir until combined, and shape the mixture into uniform balls.
3. Bake the balls on a greased baking sheet for 25 minutes at 350 degrees F until browned.
4. Meanwhile, spread sweet potatoes on a baking sheet lined with baking paper, drizzle with ½ tablespoon oil, toss until coated, and bake for 20 minutes with the meatballs.
5. Prepare the dressing, and for this, place the remaining ingredients for the salad in a food processor and pulse until smooth.
6. Place roasted sweet potatoes in a bowl, drizzle with the dressing, toss until coated, and then top with meatballs.
7. Serve straight away.

Preparation Time: 10-75 minutes
Cooking Time: 15 minutes
Servings: 4

153. Kale Slaw

INGREDIENTS:

- 1 small bunch kale, chopped
- ½ small head cabbage, shredded
- ¼ onion, thinly sliced
- ¼ cup tender herbs (cilantro, basil, parsley, chives)
- ¼ cup olive oil
- 4 tablespoons lemon juice
- 2 garlic cloves, minced
- salt, pepper, and chili flakes

DIRECTIONS:

1. Combine kale, cabbage, herbs, and onions in a large bowl.
2. Add olive oil, lemon juice, minced garlic, salt, pepper and mix well.
3. Add chili flakes, toss well before serving.

Nutrition: *Calories: 140 Cal; Fat: 0.9 g; Carbs: 27.1 g; Protein: 6.3 g; Fiber: 6.2 g*

Preparation Time: 10 minutes
Cooking Time: 20 minutes
Servings: 4

154. Chili Tofu

INGREDIENTS:

- 10 oz. firm tofu, cubed
- 1 tbsp. soy sauce
- 1 tsp. curry powder
- 1 tsp. balsamic vinegar
- 1 tbsp. fish sauce
- 1 tsp. olive oil
- 1 tsp. dried parsley
- 1 tsp. tomato paste
- 1/2 tsp. chili flakes

DIRECTION

1. In the instant pot mix the tofu with the soy sauce, curry powder and the other ingredients and toss gently.
2. After this, preheat instant pot on Sauté mode.
3. Cook the meal for 2 minutes from each side.
4. Transfer the cooked tofu in the serving bowls and let it chill to room temperature. Serve and enjoy!

Nutrition: *Calories: 183, Fat: 8.3 g, Protein: 12.8 g, Carbs: 4.7 g, Fiber: 1.4 g*

Preparation Time: 10 minutes
Cooking Time: 20 minutes
Servings: 4

155. Barbecue Mushrooms

INGREDIENTS:

- 3 pounds Trumpet mushrooms
- 2 tbsp. BBQ sauce
- 1/2 cup tomato sauce
- 1 onion, diced
- 1 tsp. sweet paprika
- 1 tsp. oregano, dried
- 1 jalapeno pepper, diced
- 1 tsp. olive oil
- 1/4 cup water

DIRECTION

1. In the instant pot mix the mushrooms with the BBQ sauce and the other ingredients and toss gently. Close and seal the lid.
2. Cook the mushrooms for 5 minutes on manual mode (high pressure).
3. Then allow natural pressure release for 5 minutes more.
4. Open the lid, mix up the meal well and transfer into the serving bowl. Serve and enjoy!

Nutrition *Calories: 187, Fat: 5.6 g, Protein: 4.1 g, Carbs: 15.3 g, Fiber: 6.1 g*

Preparation Time: **10 minutes**
Cooking Time: **30 minutes**
Servings: **3**

156. Mushrooms and Red Wine Sauce

INGREDIENTS:

- 1/2 cup red wine
- 2 cups mushrooms, chopped
- 1 tbsp. tomato paste
- 1 tsp. chili powder
- 1 tsp. coriander, ground
- 1 tbsp. Italian seasoning
- 1 cup vegetable stock
- 1/2 tsp. salt
- 1/2 tsp. black pepper
- 1/4 tsp. dried rosemary
- 1 tbsp. olive oil
- 1 onion, chopped

DIRECTION

1. In the instant pot, combine together the mushrooms with wine, tomato paste, chili powder and the other ingredients. Toss and seal the lid.
2. Cook the mixture on Sauté mode for 20 minutes.
3. When the time is over, mix up the cooked meal well and transfer into the serving bowls. Serve and enjoy!

Nutrition *Calories: 318, Fat: 7.4 g Protein: 2.3 g, Carbs: 12.7 g Fiber: 2 g*

Preparation Time: **10 minutes**
Cooking Time: **30 minutes**
Servings: **4**

157. Herbed Gnocchi

INGREDIENTS:

- 1 1/2 cup gnocchi
- 1 tbsp. fresh dill, chopped
- 1 tbsp. cilantro, chopped
- 1 tbsp. oregano, chopped
- 1 tbsp. dill, chopped
- 1 zucchini, diced
- 1 tsp. salt
- 1/2 cup almond milk
- 1/2 tsp. chili flakes
- 1/2 tsp. ground black pepper
- 1 tsp. olive oil
- 1 cup water

DIRECTION

1. Pour water in the instant pot. Add gnocchi, close and seal the lid.
2. Set Manual mode (high pressure) and cook it for 8 minutes. Make a quick pressure release.
3. Drain water and transfer gnocchi into the bowl.
4. Pour olive oil in the instant pot. Add zucchini, return the gnocchi and the other ingredients.
5. Toss and cook on Sauté mode for 10 minutes.
6. When the time is over, mix up the cooked meal well and transfer onto serving plates. Enjoy!

Nutrition: *Calories: 303, Fat: 8.8 g, Protein: 3 g, Carbs: 11.7 g, Fiber: 2.5 g*

Preparation Time: 10 minutes
Cooking Time: 15 minutes
Servings: 4

158. Popcorn Broccoli

INGREDIENTS:

- 1/2 cup broccoli florets
- 1 tsp. turmeric
- 1 tsp. curry powder
- 1/4 cup almond flour
- 4 tbsp. coconut cream
- 1 tsp. salt
- 1 tsp. black pepper
- 1 tbsp. bread crumbs
- 1 cup water, for cooking

DIRECTION

1. In the mixing bowl combine together the broccoli with turmeric and the other ingredients except bread crumbs and water and toss well.
2. Sprinkle the popcorn broccoli with the bread crumbs.
3. Pour water in the instant pot and insert rack.
4. Place popcorn into the instant pot pan.
5. Transfer the pan on the rack. Close and seal the lid.
6. Cook cauliflower popcorn for 7 minutes on manual mode (high pressure).
7. When the time is over, use quick pressure release.
8. Open the lid and chill the meal to room temperature. Serve and enjoy!

Nutrition *Calories: 153, Fat: 5.8 g, Protein: 3.5 g, Carbs: 6.7 g, Fiber: 2.4 g*

Preparation Time: 10 minutes
Cooking Time: 20 minutes
Servings: 4

159. Soy Broccoli

INGREDIENTS:

- 1 pound broccoli florets
- 1 tsp. salt
- 1 tsp. paprika
- 1/2 tsp. black pepper
- 1 tsp. chili powder
- 1/2 tsp. ground cardamom
- 1 tsp. ground black pepper
- 1 tbsp. tomato paste
- 1 tsp. soy sauce
- 1 tsp. olive oil
- 1/2 cup vegetable stock

DIRECTION

1. In the instant pot, mxi the broccoli with the salt, pepper, paprika and the other ingredients and toss. Close and seal the lid.
2. Set high-pressure mode (manual) and cook it for 5 minutes.
3. Then allow natural pressure release.
4. Open the instant pot lid and divide into bowls. Serve and enjoy!

Nutrition *Calories: 163, Fat: 5.6 g, Protein: 3.2 g, Carbs: 11.8 g, Fiber: 1.6 g*

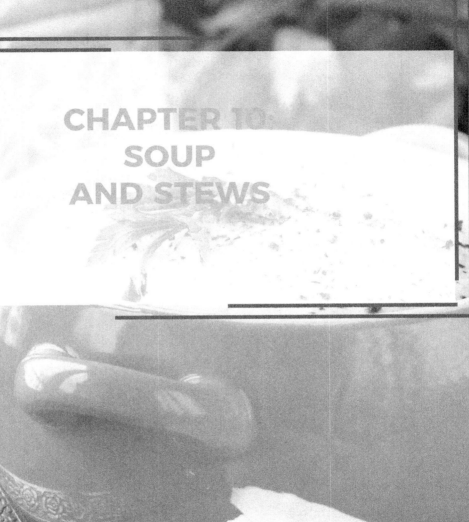

CHAPTER 10:
SOUP
AND STEWS

Preparation Time: 10 minutes
Cooking Time: 15 minutes
Servings: 4

160. Cauliflower Soup

INGREDIENTS:

- 1-pound cauliflower head
- ¼ cup coconut cream
- 2 cups of water
- 2 tablespoon lemon juice
- 1 tablespoon olive oil
- 1 onion, diced
- 1 teaspoon salt
- ½ teaspoon ground black pepper
- ½ cup water, for cooking

DIRECTIONS:

1. Pour ½ cup of water in the instant pot and insert steamer rack.
2. Place cauliflower on the rack and close the lid.
3. Cook it on Manual mode for 5 minutes. Then use quick pressure release.
4. Remove the cauliflower head from the instant pot.
5. Remove water.
6. Pour olive oil into the instant pot. Add diced onion and saute it for 4 minutes.
7. Sprinkle the onion with salt and ground black pepper.
8. Chop cooked cauliflower and add into the instant pot.
9. Then add water and coconut cream.
10. Close and seal the lid. Set Manual mode and cook the meal for 4 minutes.
11. Use quick pressure release.
12. Open the lid and blend the mixture until smooth.
13. Ladle the soup in the bowls and sprinkle with lemon juice.

Nutrition: *calories 106, fat 7.3, fiber 3.9, carbs 9.7, protein 3*

Preparation Time: 10 minutes
Cooking Time: 25 minutes
Servings: 2

161. French Onion Soup

INGREDIENTS:

- 3 cups onion, diced
- 2 tablespoons coconut oil
- ¼ cup of water
- 2 cups vegetable broth
- 1 teaspoon salt
- 1 teaspoon ground black pepper
- 1 teaspoon minced garlic
- ½ teaspoon ground nutmeg
- 3 oz vegan Parmesan, grated

Nutrition: *calories 332, fat 14, fiber 4.6, carbs 27.7, protein 19.5*

DIRECTIONS:

1. Place diced onions and coconut oil in the instant pot.
2. Set saute mode and start to cook them.
3. Sprinkle the vegetables with salt, ground black pepper, minced garlic, and ground nutmeg. Stir well.
4. When the onions start to become tender, add water and mix up the mixture well.
5. Close and seal the lid.
6. Set Manual mode (High pressure) and cook onions for 12 minutes. Then use quick pressure release.
7. Add vegetable broth and stir the soup well. Close the lid and cook on Saute mode for 10 minutes more.
8. Mix up the soup carefully and ladle into the serving bowls.
9. Top the cooked onion soup with vegan Parmesan.

Preparation Time: 10 minutes
Cooking Time: 35 minutes
Servings: 4

162. Leek Soup

INGREDIENTS:

- 3 cups leek, chopped
- 2 tablespoons coconut oil
- 1 teaspoon minced garlic
- 1 cup potatoes, chopped
- 1 tablespoon corn flour
- ½ cup coconut cream
- 3 cups of water
- ½ cup celery root, chopped
- 1 teaspoon salt
- 1 teaspoon chili flakes
- ½ teaspoon ground ginger
- ½ teaspoon white pepper
- 4 teaspoons chives, chopped

DIRECTIONS:

1. Place leek with coconut oil in the instant pot.
2. Add minced garlic, and saute the mixture for 5 minutes. Stir it from time to time.
3. When the vegetables are soft, sprinkle them with corn flour.
4. Add chopped celery root, potatoes, coconut cream, water, chili flakes, ground ginger, and white pepper.
5. Mix it up and close the lid.
6. Set Saute mode and cook soup for 30 minutes.
7. Then blend the soup until you get a creamy mixture.
8. Garnish the cooked soup with chopped chives.

Nutrition: *calories 212, fat 14.4, fiber 3.4, carbs 20.8, protein 2.9*

Preparation Time: 10 minutes
Cooking Time: 30 minutes
Servings: 4

163. Endives and Rice Soup

INGREDIENTS:

- 1 tbsp. butter
- 2 tsps. sesame oil
- 2 scallions, chopped
- 3 garlic cloves chopped
- 1 tbsp. ginger, grated
- 1 tsp. chili sauce
- A pinch of salt and black pepper
- ½ cup white rice
- 6 cups veggie stock
- 3 endives, trimmed and chopped

DIRECTIONS:

1. Melt the butter on Sauté and add the sesame oil. Add garlic, scallions, ginger, and chili sauce. Cook for 5 minutes. Add stock and rice, mix and cover.
2. Cook on High for 17 minutes. Add salt, pepper, and endives, stir, and cover. Cook on High for 5 minutes more. Serve.

Nutrition: *calories 357, fat 14.8, fiber 2.8, carbs 51.7, protein 5.8*

Preparation Time: **20 minutes**
Cooking Time: **55 minutes**
Servings: **6**

164. Creamy Sweet Potato & Coconut Curry

INGREDIENTS:

- 2 pounds of sweet potatoes, peeled and chopped
- 1/2 pound of red cabbage, shredded
- 2 red chilies, seeded and sliced
- 2 medium-sized red bell peppers, cored and sliced
- 2 large white onions, peeled and sliced
- 1 1/2 teaspoon of minced garlic
- 1 teaspoon of grated ginger
- 1/2 teaspoon of salt
- 1 teaspoon of paprika
- 1/2 teaspoon of cayenne pepper
- 2 tablespoons of peanut butter
- 4 tablespoons of olive oil
- 12-ounce of tomato puree
- 14 fluid ounce of coconut milk
- 1/2 cup of chopped coriander

DIRECTIONS:

1. Place a large non-stick skillet pan over an average heat, add 1 tablespoon of oil and let it heat.
2. Then add the onion and cook for 10 minutes or until it gets soft.
3. Add the garlic, ginger, salt, paprika, cayenne pepper and continue cooking for 2 minutes or until it starts producing fragrance.
4. Transfer this mixture to a 6-quarts slow cooker, and reserve the pan.
5. In the pan, add 1 tablespoon of oil and let it heat.
6. Add the cabbage, red chili, bell pepper and cook it for 5 minutes.
7. Then transfer this mixture to the slow cooker and reserve the pan.
8. Add the remaining oil to the pan; the sweet potatoes in a single layer and cook it in 3 batches for 5 minutes or until it starts getting brown.
9. Add the sweet potatoes to the slow cooker, along with tomato puree, coconut milk and stir properly.
10. Cover the top, plug in the slow cooker; adjust the cooking time to 6 hours and let it cook on the low heat setting or until the sweet potatoes are tender.
11. When done, add the seasoning and pour it in the peanut butter.
12. Garnish it with coriander and serve.

Nutrition: *calories 108, fat 50, fiber 2, carbs 8, protein 48*

Preparation Time: 10 minutes
Cooking Time: 30 minutes
Servings: 4

165. Lentil Curry

INGREDIENTS:

- 1½ cups lentils, rinsed
- 1 tbsp. garlic, minced
- 1½ tbsps. lemon juice
- 1½ tbsps. ginger, minced
- 4 cups of water
- 1½ tsps. salt
- 1½ tsps. cumin seeds
- 3 medium tomatoes, chopped
- 1½ tbsp. oil
- 2 medium onions, diced
- Cilantro, to garnish

DIRECTIONS:

1. Add the oil, cumin, garlic, and onions in the Instant Pot and cook on Sauté for 4 minutes. Add rest of the ingredients except for lime juice and cilantro. Cover and cook on High for 15 minutes. Do a quick release. Open and add lime juice and cilantro. Serve.

Nutrition: *calories 357, fat 14.8, fiber 2.8, carbs 51.7, protein 5.8*

Preparation Time: 10 minutes
Cooking Time: 30 minutes
Servings: 4

166. Kidney Bean Curry

INGREDIENTS:

- 1 cup dried red kidney beans, soaked for overnight and drained
- ¼ cup split chickpeas, soaked for overnight and drained
- 4 cups of water
- 3 tbsps. olive oil
- 3 tsps. garlic, minced
- 1 large tomato, chopped finely
- 2 medium onions, chopped
- 3 tsps. fresh ginger, minced
- 1½ tsps. ground coriander
- 1½ tsps. ground turmeric
- 1½ tsps. ground cumin
- 2 tsps. red chili powder
- ¼ tsp. salt
- 4 tbsps. fresh cilantro, chopped

DIRECTIONS:

1. Put the oil, garlic, ginger, and onions in the pot and press Sauté. Sauté for 4 minutes. Add coriander, turmeric, cumin, red chili powder, and salt. Sauté for 4 minutes. Add water, tomatoes, beans, and chickpeas. Cover and cook on High for 20 minutes. Open, garnish, and serve.

Nutrition: *calories 347, fat 14.8, fiber 2.8, carbs 51.7, protein 5.8*

Preparation Time: 10 minutes
Cooking Time: 30 minutes
Servings: 4

167. Spinach Curry

INGREDIENTS:

- 1 tsp. butter
- 1/3 cup brown lentils
- 1 small ginger piece, grated
- 4 garlic cloves, minced
- 1 green chili pepper, chopped
- 2 tomatoes, chopped
- ½ tsp. garam masala
- ½ tsp. turmeric powder
- 2 potatoes, cubed
- A pinch of salt and black pepper
- ¼ tsp. cardamom, ground
- ¼ tsp. cinnamon powder
- 1 cup of water
- 6 ounces of spinach leaves

DIRECTIONS:

1. Melt the butter on Sauté. Add chili pepper, ginger, and garlic. Cook for 3 minutes. Add tomatoes, salt, pepper, cinnamon, cardamom, turmeric, and garam masala. Cook for 4 minutes. Add lentils, potatoes, water, and spinach.
2. Cover and cook on High for 8 minutes. Open and serve.

Nutrition: *Calories 210; Carbs 36g; Fat 5g; Protein 10g*

Preparation Time: 10 minutes
Cooking Time: 7 minutes
Servings: 4

168. Noodle Soup

INGREDIENTS:

- ¼ teaspoon fresh ginger, grated
- 1 teaspoon salt
- ½ teaspoon ground black pepper
- 4 cups of water
- 5 oz noodles, cooked
- 4 oz celery stalk, chopped
- 1 teaspoon garlic powder
- 1 cup baby carrots
- 1 teaspoon sesame oil

DIRECTIONS:

1. Preheat instant pot on Saute mode and pour sesame oil.
2. Add chopped celery stalk and saute it for 2-3 minutes.
3. Meanwhile, cut baby carrots into the halves. Add them in the instant pot too
4. Sprinkle the ingredients with salt, ground black pepper, and garlic powder.
5. Then add water and grated ginger.
6. Close and seal the lid. Set Manual mode (High pressure) and cook soup for 4 minutes
7. Then use quick pressure release.
8. Add cooked noodles, mix up soup well and ladle into the bowls.

Nutrition: *calories 82, fat 1.9, fiber 2, carbs 14, protein 2.5*

Preparation Time: 10 minutes
Cooking Time: 20 minutes
Servings: 4

169. Sweet Potato Stew

INGREDIENTS:

- 1 small yellow onion, chopped
- 1 tbsp. butter
- 2 garlic cloves, minced
- A small ginger piece, grated
- 2 sweet potatoes, chopped
- 1 zucchini, chopped
- 1 red bell pepper, chopped
- 14 ounces canned tomatoes, chopped
- 1 tsp. turmeric powder
- 2 tsps. curry powder
- A pinch of salt and black pepper
- 2 tbsps. red curry paste
- 14 ounces milk
- Juice from 3 limes
- 1 tbsp. cilantro, chopped

DIRECTIONS:

1. Melt the butter on Sauté. Add onion and cook for 3 minutes. Add garlic and ginger and cook for 1 minute more.
2. Add sweet potatoes, zucchini, bell pepper, tomatoes, turmeric, curry powder, curry paste, salt, pepper, milk, and cover. Cook on High for 5 minutes.
3. Add lime juice and cilantro. Serve.

Nutrition: *Calories 300; Carbs 12g; Fat 9g; Protein 7g*

Preparation Time: 10 minutes
Cooking Time: 30 minutes
Servings: 4

170. Split Pea Stew

INGREDIENTS:

- 1 carrot, cubed
- 1 yellow onion, chopped
- 1 and ½ tbsps. butter
- 1 celery stick, chopped
- 5 garlic cloves, minced
- 1 bay leaf
- 1 and ½ tsp.. cumin, ground
- 1 tsp. sweet paprika
- ¼ tsp. chili powder
- A pinch of salt and black pepper
- ¼ tsp. cinnamon powder
- ½ cup tomatoes, chopped
- Juice of ½ lemon
- 2 cups yellow peas
- 1-quart veggie stock
- 1 tbsp. chives, chopped

DIRECTIONS:

1. Melt the butter on Sauté. Add carrots, onion, and celery and cook for 4 minutes.
2. Add the garlic, bay leaf, cumin, paprika, chili powder, salt, pepper, cinnamon, tomatoes, lemon juice, peas, and stock. Cover and cook on High for 10 minutes. Open and add chives. Mix and serve.

Nutrition: *Calories 312; Carbs 12g; Fat 6g; Protein 7g*

Preparation Time: 15 minutes
Cooking Time: 25 minutes
Serving: 4

171. Mushroom Curry

INGREDIENTS:

- 2 cups plum tomatoes, chopped
- 2 tablespoons grapeseed oil
- 1 small onion, chopped finely
- ¼ teaspoon cayenne powder
- 4 cups fresh button mushrooms, sliced
- 1¼ cups spring water
- ¼ cup unsweetened coconut milk
- Sea salt, as required

DIRECTIONS:

1. In a food processor, add the tomatoes and pulse until a smooth paste form. In a pan, heat the oil over medium heat and sauté the onion for about 5-6 minutes.
2. Add the tomato paste and cook for about 5 minutes. Stir in the mushrooms, water and coconut milk and bring to a boil. Cook for about 10-12 minutes, stirring occasionally. Season it well and remove from the heat. Serve hot.

Nutrition: *calories 280, fat 8, fiber 3, carbs 8, protein 6*

Preparation Time: 5 minutes
Cooking Time: 12 minutes
Servings: 6

172. Cream of Mushroom Soup

INGREDIENTS:

- 1 medium white onion, peeled, chopped
- 16 ounces button mushrooms, sliced
- 1 ½ teaspoon minced garlic
- 1/4 cup all-purpose flour
- 1/2 teaspoon ground black pepper
- 1 teaspoon dried thyme
- 1/4 teaspoon nutmeg
- 1/2 teaspoon salt
- 2 tablespoons vegan butter
- 4 cups vegetable broth
- 1 1/2 cups coconut milk, unsweetened

DIRECTIONS:

1. Take a large pot, place it over medium-high heat, add butter and when it melts, add onions and garlic, stir in garlic and cook for 5 minutes until softened and nicely brown.
2. Then sprinkle flour over vegetables, continue cooking for 1 minute, then add remaining ingredients, stir until mixed and simmer for 5 minutes until thickened.
3. Serve straight away

Nutrition: *Calories: 120 Cal Fat: 7 g Carbs: 10 g Protein: 2 g Fiber: 6 g*

Preparation Time: 10 minutes
Cooking Time: 6 hours
Servings: 6

173. Black Bean and Quinoa Stew

INGREDIENTS:

- 1 pound black beans, dried, soaked overnight
- 3/4 cup quinoa, uncooked
- 1 medium red bell pepper, cored, chopped
- 1 medium red onion, peeled, diced
- 1 medium green bell pepper, cored, chopped
- 28-ounce diced tomatoes
- 2 dried chipotle peppers
- 1 ½ teaspoon minced garlic
- 2/3 teaspoon sea salt
- 2 teaspoons red chili powder
- 1/3 teaspoon ground black pepper
- 1 teaspoon coriander powder
- 1 dried cinnamon stick
- 1/4 cup cilantro
- 7 cups of water

DIRECTIONS:

1. Switch on the slow cooker, add all the ingredients in it, except for salt, and stir until mixed.
2. Shut the cooker with lid and cook for 6 hours at a high heat setting until cooked.
3. When done, stir salt into the stew until mixed, remove cinnamon sticks and serve.

Nutrition: *Calories: 308 Cal Fat: 2 g Carbs: 70 g Protein: 23 g Fiber: 32 g*

Preparation Time: 5 minutes
Cooking Time: 40 minutes
Servings: 4

174. Creamy Artichoke Soup

INGREDIENTS:

- 1 can artichoke hearts, drained
- 3 cups vegetable broth
- 2 tablespoon lemon juice
- 1 small onion, finely cut
- 2 cloves garlic, crushed
- 3 tablespoon olive oil
- 2 tablespoon flour
- 1/2 cup vegan cream

DIRECTIONS:

1. Gently sauté the onion and garlic in some olive oil.
2. Add the flour, whisking constantly, and then add the hot vegetable broth slowly, while still whisking. Cook for about 5 minutes.
3. Blend the artichoke, lemon juice, salt and pepper until smooth. Add the puree to the broth mix, stir well, and then stir in the cream.
4. Cook until heated through. Garnish with a swirl of vegan cream or a sliver of artichoke.

Nutrition: *Calories: 211; Carbs: 12g; Fat: 7g; Protein: 11g*

Preparation Time: 5 minutes
Cooking Time: 35 minutes
Servings: 4

175. Tomato Artichoke Soup

INGREDIENTS:

- 1 can artichoke hearts, drained
- 1 can diced tomatoes, undrained
- 3 cups vegetable broth
- 1 small onion, chopped
- 2 cloves garlic, crushed
- 1 tablespoon pesto
- Black pepper, to taste

DIRECTIONS:

1. Combine all Ingredients: in the slow cooker.
2. Cover and cook on low for 8-10 hours or on high for 4-5 hours.
3. Blend the soup in batches and return it to the slow cooker. Season with salt and pepper to taste and serve.

Nutrition: *Calories: 211; Carbs: 10g; Fat: 7g; Protein: 11g*

Preparation Time: 10 minutes
Cooking Time: 50 minutes
Servings: 4

176. Lasagna Soup

INGREDIENTS:

- 8 lasagna noodles (gluten-free and uncooked)
- 1 block of tofu (firm and crumbled)
- 6 cups of vegetable broth
- 1 can of tomatoes (crushed)
- 4 garlic cloves (minced)
- 1 onion (diced)
- 2 tbsp of olive oil
- 2 tbsp of nutritional yeast
- 1 tbsp of low-sodium soy sauce
- 1 tsp of sweet basil
- 1 tsp of red chili flakes
- ½ tsp of onion powder
- ½ tsp of black pepper
- Toppings: Vegan mozzarella (grated)

DIRECTIONS:

1. Set the oven to 350 degrees-Fahrenheit. Prep a baking sheet with a single layer of parchment paper.
2. Mix the soy sauce, red chili flakes, 1 tbsp olive oil, nutritional yeast, and onion powder in a bowl to form a paste-like mixture.
3. Crumble the tofu and mix it into the seasoning to marinate in the sauce. Spread the tofu in a large pan, and bake it for 40 minutes while stirring it regularly.
4. Bring a soup pot to high heat, adding 1 tbsp of olive oil to the pot. Add the diced onion and minced garlic to the pot and cook it for 5 minutes.
5. Add the vegetable broth, tomatoes, and sweet basil to the pot, and allow it to cook for 10 minutes. Once done, add the noodles to the pot. Cook it for 10 minutes. Stir the soup regularly.
6. Add in the tofu and cook the soup for 1 more minute. Depending on your desired consistency, you can add water as needed. However, the consistency is adequate to make a thick soup.
7. Serve the soup hot immediately, topping it with grated vegan mozzarella cheese, or store it in large airtight mason jars for up to 3 days.

Nutrition: *Calories: 310, Carbohydrates: 49g, Protein: 14g, Fat: 7g*

Preparation Time: 5 minutes
Cooking Time: 15 minutes
Servings: 4

177. Potato Cream Soup

INGREDIENTS:

- 1 cup of coconut milk
- 2 cups of water
- 2 cups potatoes, chopped
- 1 onion, sliced
- 1 teaspoon turmeric
- 1 teaspoon salt
- 1 tablespoon avocado oil
- 1 teaspoon chili flakes
- ½ cup fresh cilantro, chopped

DIRECTIONS:

1. Pour avocado oil in the instant pot and pre-heat it on Saute mode.
2. When the oil is hot, add sliced onion and chopped potatoes.
3. Sprinkle the vegetables with turmeric, salt, and chili flakes. Mix up the ingredients and saute for 5 minutes.
4. Then add coconut milk and water. Close and seal the lid.
5. Cook soup on Manual mode for 10 minutes. Then use quick pressure release.
6. Open the lid and blend soup with the help of the hand blender.
7. When the liquid is smooth, transfer it into the serving bowls.
8. Sprinkle the soup with cilantro before serving.

Nutrition: *calories 208, fat 14.9, fiber 4.1, carbs 18.3, protein 3.1*

Preparation Time: 5 minutes
Cooking Time: 15 minutes
Servings: 3

178. Quinoa Tomato Soup

INGREDIENTS:

- 1 carrot, diced
- ½ onion, diced
- 1 cup quinoa
- 1 cup tomato puree
- 1 tablespoon fresh dill
- ½ bell pepper, chopped
- 1 cup of water
- 1 teaspoon salt
- 1 teaspoon cayenne pepper
- 1/3 cup green peas
- 1 teaspoon almond butter

DIRECTIONS:

1. Toss butter in the instant pot and melt it on Saute mode.
2. Add carrot, onion, and bell pepper. Saute the ingredients for 10 minutes. Mix p them from time to time.
3. After this, add quinoa, green peas, cayenne pepper, salt, fresh dill, and water.
4. Add tomato puree, mix up the soup and close the lid.
5. Set Manual (high pressure) mode and cook soup for 3 minutes.
6. Then use quick pressure release.
7. Mix up the cooked soup well before serving.

Nutrition: *calories 313, fat 6.9, fiber 8.4, carbs 53.3, protein 12.2*

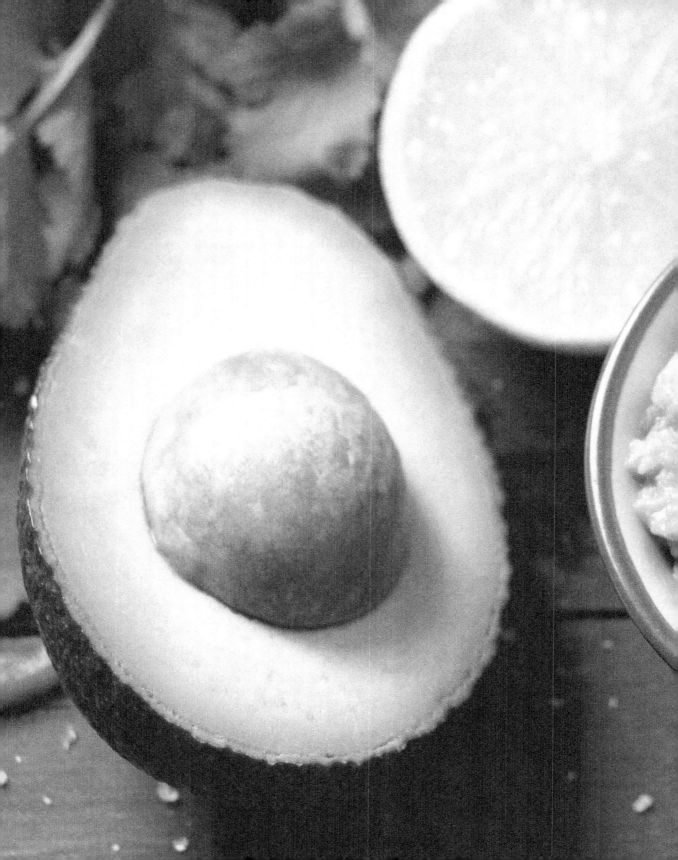

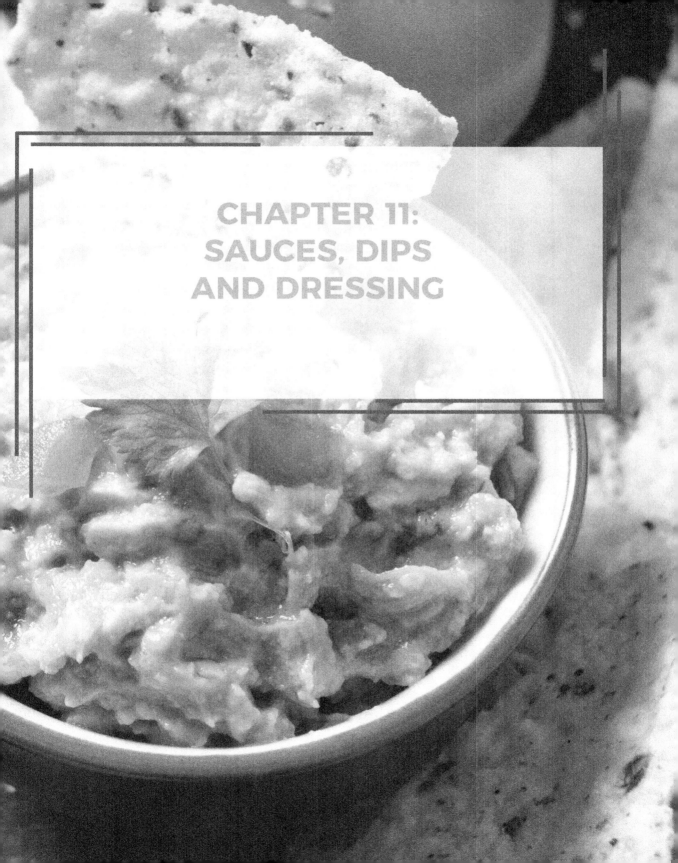

CHAPTER 11:
SAUCES, DIPS AND DRESSING

Preparation Time: 10 minutes
Cooking Time: 5 minutes
Servings: 7

179. Avocado Pesto

INGREDIENTS:

- 2 cups spinach, chopped
- 1 tablespoon olive oil
- 1 teaspoon minced garlic
- 1 tablespoon fresh basil
- 1 tablespoon lemon juice
- 1 avocado, peeled, chopped
- ¼ cup sesame oil
- 1 teaspoon salt
- ½ teaspoon cayenne pepper

DIRECTIONS:

1. Place chopped spinach and olive oil in the instant pot.
2. Add lemon juice and salt. Stir well.
3. Cook the greens on saute mode for 5 minutes.
4. Transfer the cooked spinach in the blender.
5. Add minced garlic, fresh basil, avocado, sesame oil, and cayenne pepper.
6. Blend the mixture until smooth.
7. Pour the cooked pesto sauce in the sauce bowl.

Nutrition: *calories 148, fat 15.5, fiber 2.2, carbs 3, protein 0.9*

Preparation Time: 10 minutes
Cooking Time: 2 minutes
Servings: 6

180. Basil Cream Sauce

INGREDIENTS:

- 1 cup coconut cream
- ½ cup of water
- 1 cup fresh basil, chopped
- 1 garlic clove, peeled
- 1 teaspoon salt
- 1 teaspoon Italian spices
- 1 teaspoon nutritional yeasts

DIRECTIONS:

1. Place fresh basil in the instant pot.
2. Add water and coconut cream.
3. Sprinkle the greens with salt and Italian seasoning.
4. Close and seal the lid.
5. Cook basil for 2 minutes on high-pressure mode. Use quick pressure release.
6. Open the lid and add garlic clove. Blend the mixture until smooth.
7. When the mixture gets to room temperature, add nutritional yeast and mix up well.
8. Transfer the sauce in the serving bowl

Nutrition: *calories 96, fat 9.6, fiber 1.1, carbs 2.8, protein 1.3*

Preparation Time: 10 minutes
Cooking Time: 5 minutes
Servings: 3

181. Cacao Spread

INGREDIENTS:

- 1 tablespoon nuts
- ½ cup cashew milk
- 1 tablespoon raw cacao powder
- ¼ cup of sugar
- 1 teaspoon almond butter

DIRECTIONS:

1. Blend together raw cacao powder and cashew milk.
2. Pour the liquid in the instant pot.
3. Add sugar and almond butter.
4. Cook the mixture on Saute mode for 5 minutes. Stir it from time to time.
5. Add nuts and mix up well.
6. Close the lid. Switch off the instant pot and let it rest for 10 minutes.

Nutrition: *calories 142, fat 5.3, fiber 2.6, carbs 22.9, protein 2.5*

Preparation Time: 5 minutes
Cooking Time: 3 hours
Servings: 6

182. Caramel Pumpkin Sauce

INGREDIENTS:

- 6 oz pumpkin puree
- 8 oz almond milk
- 1 cup of sugar
- 1 teaspoon ground cinnamon
- 1 teaspoon coconut oil

DIRECTIONS:

1. Put all the ingredients in the instant pot and mix up them well.
2. Close the lid and cook the sauce on Low-pressure mode for 3 hours.

Nutrition: *calories 229, fat 9.9, fiber 1.9, carbs 38, protein 1.2*

Preparation Time: 10 minutes
Cooking Time: 10 minutes
Servings: 3

183. Cauliflower Sauce

INGREDIENTS:

- 7 oz cauliflower
- 1 cup of water
- ½ cup almond milk
- 1 teaspoon salt
- 1 teaspoon ground black pepper
- 1 tablespoon wheat flour

DIRECTIONS:

1. Place cauliflower and water in the instant pot.
2. Close and seal the lid. Cook the vegetable on Manual mode (high pressure) for 7 minutes.
3. Then make quick pressure release and open the lid.
4. Drain the water and mash cauliflower with the help of the fork
5. Add salt, ground black pepper, wheat flour, and almond milk.
6. Mix up the mixture well.
7. Cook it on Saute mode for 3 minutes more.
8. The cooked sauce shouldn't be smooth.

Nutrition: *calories 120, fat 9.7, fiber 2.8, carbs 8.2, protein 2.6*

Preparation Time: 5 minutes
Cooking Time: 15 minutes
Servings: 2

184. Cayenne Pepper Filling

INGREDIENTS:

- 1 sweet potato, peeled, chopped
- 1 cayenne pepper, chopped
- ½ cup of water
- 1 tablespoon almond yogurt
- 1 teaspoon olive oil
- 1 carrot, grated
- 1 teaspoon mustard

DIRECTIONS:

1. Pour olive oil in the instant pot and preheat it on Saute mode.
2. Add chopped sweet potato and cayenne pepper.
3. Saute the vegetables for 5 minutes.
4. Add grated carrot and stir it well.
5. Then pour water in the instant pot and add mustard and almond yogurt. Mix up the mixture.
6. Close and seal the lid.
7. Cook the filling on Manual mode (high pressure) for 5 minutes. Then make a quick pressure release and transfer the meal in the serving plate.

Nutrition: *calories 103, fat 3.2, fiber 3.5, carbs 17, protein 1.9*

Preparation Time: 10 minutes
Cooking Time: 2 minutes
Servings: 6

185. Cranberry Sauce

INGREDIENTS:

- 8 oz cranberries
- 3 oz maple syrup
- 1 tablespoon lemon juice
- ¾ teaspoon dried oregano

DIRECTIONS:

1. Place cranberries, maple syrup, lemon juice, and dried oregano in the instant pot. Stir gently.
2. Close and seal the lid.
3. Cook the sauce on manual mode for 2 minutes. When the time is over, allow natural pressure release for 5 minutes more.
4. Stir the sauce gently before serving.

Nutrition: *calories 59, fat 0.1, fiber 1.5, carbs 13.1, protein 0*

Preparation Time: 10 minutes
Cooking Time: 5 minutes
Servings: 4

186. Creamy Green Peas Filling

INGREDIENTS:

- 2 cups green peas, frozen
- 2 cups of water
- ½ cup coconut cream
- 1 teaspoon tahini paste
- 1 oz fresh dill, chopped

DIRECTIONS:

1. Place green peas and water in the instant pot.
2. Close and seal the lid. Cook green peas for 5 minutes on manual mode.
3. After this, use quick pressure release.
4. Open the lid and drain the water.
5. Then transfer the green peas in the food processor.
6. Add coconut cream, tahini paste, and chopped dill. Blend it until homogenous.
7. Store the filling in the closed container in the fridge up to 4 days.

Nutrition: *calories 153, fat 8.4, fiber 5.4, carbs 16.4, protein 6.3*

Preparation Time: 10 minutes
Cooking Time: 4 minutes
Servings: 6

187. Mexican Rice Filling

INGREDIENTS:

- ½ cup black beans, canned
- 2 cups of water
- 1 cup fresh cilantro, chopped
- ½ cup corn kernels, frozen
- 1 cup of rice
- 1 teaspoon salt
- 1 tablespoon olive oil
- ½ teaspoon paprika
- 1 teaspoon chili flakes

DIRECTIONS:

1. Place rice and water in the instant pot. Add salt and corn kernels.
2. Close and seal the lid. Set rice mode (high pressure) and cook rice for 4 minutes. Use quick pressure release.
3. Meanwhile, in the mixing bowl mix up together canned black beans, olive oil, paprika, chili flakes, and chopped cilantro. Mix up the mixture well.
4. When the rice and corn are cooked, chill them to the room temperature and add in the beans mixture. Mix up well.

Nutrition: *calories 200, fat 2.9, fiber 3.4, carbs 37.4, protein 6.2*

Preparation Time: 5 minutes
Cooking Time: 4 minutes
Servings: 4

188. Mushroom Sauce

INGREDIENTS:

- 1 cup mushrooms, grinded
- 1 onion, grinded
- 1 cup of coconut milk
- 1 teaspoon salt
- 1 teaspoon white pepper
- ¼ teaspoon ground thyme

DIRECTIONS:

1. Place grinded mushrooms and onion in the instant pot.
2. Add salt, white pepper, and ground thyme.
3. After this, add coconut milk and mix up the mixture well.
4. Close the lid and set manual mode. Cook the sauce for 4 minutes.
5. Then use quick pressure release.
6. Open the lid and mix up the cooked sauce well.

Nutrition: *calories 154, fat 14.4, fiber 2.3, carbs 6.9, protein 2.3*

Preparation Time: 15 minutes
Cooking Time: 10 minutes
Servings: 4

189. Pear Filling

INGREDIENTS:

- 2 cups pears, chopped
- 1 teaspoon ground cinnamon
- ½ teaspoon ground clove
- 1 tablespoon maple syrup
- 2 tablespoons brown sugar

DIRECTIONS:

1. Place pears in the instant pot.
2. Sprinkle them with ground cinnamon, clove, maple syrup, and brown sugar.
3. Mix up the fruits well and let them rest for 5-10 minutes or until they start to give juice.
4. After this, cook filling on Saute mode for 10 minutes. Stir it from time to time.
5. Chill the filling well.

Nutrition: *calories 79, fat 0.2, fiber 2.9, carbs 20.7, protein 0.3*

Preparation Time: 5 minutes
Cooking Time: 3 minutes
Servings: 4

190. Queso Sauce

INGREDIENTS:

- ½ can chilies, chopped, drained
- 6 oz cashew
- ½ teaspoon taco seasoning
- ½ red onion, diced
- 1 teaspoon olive oil
- 1 teaspoon paprika
- ¼ cup of water

DIRECTIONS:

1. Pour olive oil in the instant pot.
2. Set Saute mode and preheat it.
3. Add red onion and saute it until it is soft.
4. Then transfer the cooked onion in the food processor.
5. Add cashew, chopped chilies, paprika, water, and taco seasoning.
6. Blend the mixture until you get a smooth sauce.
7. Store the sauce in the fridge in the closed container up to 2 days.

Nutrition: *calories 265, fat 21, fiber 1.9, carbs 16.4, protein 6.8*

Preparation Time: 10 minutes
Cooking Time: 18 minutes
Servings: 5

191. Ravioli Sauce

INGREDIENTS:

- 1 cup tomatoes, canned, chopped
- ½ cup tomato juice
- 2 tablespoons almond yogurt
- 1 teaspoon chili pepper
- 1 teaspoon chili flakes
- 1 teaspoon salt
- ½ teaspoon paprika
- ½ teaspoon ground oregano
- ½ teaspoon ground ginger
- 1 onion, diced
- 1 teaspoon olive oil

DIRECTIONS:

1. Preheat instant pot on Saute mode.
2. Add olive oil and diced onion. Saute it for 3 minutes.
3. After this, add chopped canned tomatoes, tomato juice, chili pepper, chili flakes, salt, paprika, ground oregano, ground ginger, and stir the sauce well.
4. Close the lid and cook it on Saute mode for 15 minutes.
5. Then switch off the instant pot, add almond yogurt, mix it up, and chill the sauce till the room temperature.

Nutrition: *calories 34, fat 1.3, fiber 1.3, carbs 5.4, protein 0.9*

Preparation Time: 10 minutes
Cooking Time: 35 minutes
Servings: 4

192. Red Kidney Beans Sauce

INGREDIENTS:

- ½ cup red kidney beans, soaked
- 2 cups of water
- 1 tablespoon tomato paste
- 1 bell pepper, chopped
- 1 teaspoon salt
- 1 teaspoon chili flakes
- ½ teaspoon white pepper
- 1 tablespoon corn flour
- ¼ cup fresh dill, chopped

DIRECTIONS:

1. In the instant pot, combine together red kidney beans, water, tomato paste, chopped bell pepper, salt, chili flakes, white pepper, and dill.
2. Mix up the mixture well.
3. Close and seal the instant pot lid.
4. Set manual mode and cook the ingredients for 30 minutes.
5. Then use quick pressure release and open the lid.
6. Add corn flour and mix up the sauce well.
7. Close the lid.
8. Saute the sauce for 5 minutes on Saute mode.
9. Then stir it well and let chill till the room temperature.

Nutrition: *calories 105, fat 0.6, fiber 4.7, carbs 20.4, protein 6.4*

Preparation Time: **10 minutes**
Cooking Time: **30 minutes**
Servings: **4**

193. Artichokes Dip

INGREDIENTS:

- 1/2 lemon juice
- 1 cup water
- 1/2 cup cannellini beans, soaked for 12 hours, drained
- 2 garlic cloves, minced
- 1 pound baby artichokes, trimmed and stems cut off
- 1 cup coconut cream
- A pinch salt and black pepper

DIRECTION

1. In your instant pot, mix beans with artichokes, water, salt and pepper.
2. Stir, cover and cook on High for 20 minutes.
3. Add garlic and cream. Pulse using an immersion blender.
4. Divide into bowls. Serve and enjoy!

Nutrition: *calories 468, fat 26, fiber 8.2, carbs 56.2, protein 10.1*

Preparation Time: **20 minutes**
Cooking Time: **30 minutes**
Servings: **6**

194. Samosa Filling

INGREDIENTS:

- 1 cup chickpeas, soaked
- 3 cups of water
- 1 oz beetroot, chopped
- 1 garlic clove
- 1 tablespoon tahini paste
- 1 teaspoon salt
- ½ teaspoon harissa
- 2 tablespoons olive oil

DIRECTIONS:

1. Place the soaked chickpeas and water in the instant pot.
2. Ad beetroot and garlic clove.
3. Close and seal the lid. Cook the ingredients for 30 minutes on manual mode (high pressure). After this, allow natural pressure release for 10 minutes.
4. Place 4 tablespoons of the liquid from cooked chickpeas in the blender.
5. Add cooked chickpeas, garlic clove, and beetroot.
6. Blend the mixture until smooth.
7. Add tahini paste, salt, harissa, and olive oil. Blend the mixture well.

Nutrition: *calories 180, fat 8.1, fiber 6.1, carbs 21.6, protein 7*

Preparation Time: 10 minutes
Cooking Time: 10 minutes
Servings: 4

195. Spinach Dip

INGREDIENTS:

- 1 teaspoon onion powder
- 2 cups spinach, chopped
- ½ cup artichoke hearts, canned, chopped
- 1 tablespoon olive oil
- 1 teaspoon ground black pepper
- 1 teaspoon salt
- ½ cup of coconut yogurt
- 1 teaspoon cornstarch
- 4 oz vegan Parmesan, grated

DIRECTIONS:

1. Preheat the instant pot on Saute mode.
2. Then pour olive oil inside.
3. Add chopped spinach and chopped artichoke hearts.
4. Sprinkle the greens with ground black pepper and salt. Stir it well.
5. Close the lid and cook on Saute mode for 5 minutes.
6. After this, add coconut yogurt, onion powder, and cornstarch.
7. Add grated Parmesan and mix up the mixture well.
8. Cook it for 5 minutes more.

Nutrition: *calories 150, fat 4.1, fiber 1.6, carbs 11.5, protein 13.3*

Preparation Time: 10 minutes
Cooking Time: 6 minutes
Servings: 4

196. Vegan Cheese Sauce

INGREDIENTS:

- 1 white potato, peeled, chopped
- 1 sweet potato, peeled, chopped
- 1 carrot, chopped
- ½ cup peanuts, chopped
- 1 tablespoon lime juice
- 1 teaspoon salt
- 1 teaspoon onion powder
- 1 teaspoon ground black pepper
- 1 teaspoon chili flakes
- ½ teaspoon dried oregano
- 1 teaspoon dried basil
- 1 ½ cup water
- 1 tablespoon apple cider vinegar
- ¾ cup of coconut milk
- 1 teaspoon nutritional yeast

DIRECTIONS:

1. Put in the instant pot: chopped white potato, sweet potato, carrot, and peanuts.
2. Add water. Close and seal the lid.
3. Cook the vegetables on manual mode (high pressure) for 6 minutes.
4. Then allow natural pressure release.
5. Open the lid. Transfer the contents of the instant pot in the food processor.
6. Add lime juice, salt, onion powder, ground black pepper, chili flakes, dried oregano, dried basil, apple cider vinegar, coconut milk, and nutritional yeast.
7. Blend the mixture until smooth and homogenous.
8. Transfer the cooked cheese sauce in the serving bowl.

Nutrition: *calories 280, fat 19.9, fiber 5.3, carbs 21.9, protein 7.9*

Preparation Time: 10 minutes
Cooking Time: 6 minutes
Servings: 5

197. Vegan French Sauce

INGREDIENTS:

- 1 cup mushrooms, chopped
- ½ cup vegetable stock
- 1 teaspoon salt
- 4 oz firm tofu
- 1 tablespoon olive oil
- 1 teaspoon ground black pepper
- 1 tablespoon almond yogurt
- 1 teaspoon potato starch

DIRECTIONS:

1. Pour vegetable stock in the instant pot.
2. Add mushrooms, salt, tofu, olive oil, ground black pepper, almond yogurt, and close the lid.
3. Cook the dip on manual mode (high pressure) for 6 minutes.
4. Then make quick pressure release.
5. Open the lid and add potato starch.
6. Blend the mixture with the help of the hand blender until smooth. The sauce is cooked.

Nutrition: *calories 51, fat 4.3, fiber 0.5, carbs 2.4, protein 2.4*

Preparation Time: 10 minutes
Cooking Time: 35 minutes
Servings: 4

198. White Bean Sauce

INGREDIENTS:

- ½ cup white beans, soaked
- 1 ½ cup water
- ½ cup almond milk
- 1 tablespoon smoked paprika
- 1 teaspoon salt
- 1 cup fresh parsley, chopped
- 5 oz vegan Parmesan, grated

DIRECTIONS:

1. Place white beans, water, almond milk, smoked paprika, salt, and chopped parsley in the instant pot.
2. Close and seal the lid.
3. Cook the beans on Manual mode (high pressure) for 35 minutes.
4. Then use the quick pressure release.
5. Open the lid and add grated cheese. Mix up the sauce well until cheese is melted.

Nutrition: *calories 272, fat 7.7, fiber 5.7, carbs 26, protein 21.8*

Preparation Time: 10 minutes
Cooking Time: 12 minutes
Servings: 4

199. Mushrooms Salsa

INGREDIENTS:

- 1 tablespoon olive oil
- 1 cup cherry tomatoes, halved
- 1 avocado, peeled, pitted and cubed
- 1 tablespoon chives, chopped
- 1 small yellow onion, chopped
- 2 pounds button mushrooms, sliced
- 3 garlic cloves, minced
- 2 cups chopped spinach
- Salt and black pepper to the taste
- ¼ cup chopped parsley

DIRECTIONS:

1. Heat up a pan with the oil over medium heat, add the garlic and onion and cook for 2 minutes.
2. Add the mushrooms and the other ingredients, cook for 10 minutes more, divide into bowls and serve.

Nutrition: *calories 240, fat 8, fiber 5, carbs 10.1, protein 6.9*

Preparation Time: 10 minutes
Cooking Time: 0 minutes
Servings: 4

200. Avocado Dip

INGREDIENTS:

- 2 avocados, peeled, pitted, chopped
- Salt and black pepper to the taste
- 1 tablespoon olive oil
- 1 teaspoon mint, dried
- 1 teaspoon curry powder
- 1 tablespoon green curry paste
- 4 garlic cloves, chopped
- ½ cup tahini
- 2 tablespoons lemon juice

DIRECTIONS:

1. In a blender, mix the avocado with salt, pepper, the oil and the other ingredients.
2. Pulse until smooth then divide into bowls and serve as a snack.

Nutrition: *calories 200, fat 6.3, fiber 4.3, carbs 9, protein 7.6*

201. Tahini Dip

INGREDIENTS:

- 1 cup tahini sesame seed paste
- ½ cup coconut cream
- Salt and black pepper to the taste
- ½ cup lemon juice
- 1 tablespoon chopped cilantro
- 1 tablespoon chopped chives, chopped
- 1 teaspoon curry powder
- ½ teaspoon ground cumin
- 3 garlic cloves, chopped

DIRECTIONS:

1. In a blender, mix the tahini paste with the cream and the other ingredients, blend well, divide into bowls and serve.

Nutrition: *calories 220, fat 12, fiber 4.5, carbs 11, protein 7.1*

202. Eggplant Spread

INGREDIENTS:

- 2 pounds eggplant, baked, peeled and chopped
- A pinch of salt and black pepper
- 4 tablespoons avocado oil
- 4 garlic cloves, chopped
- Juice of 1 lemon
- Zest of 1 lemon, grated
- 1 teaspoon oregano, dried
- 1 teaspoon basil, dried
- ¼ cup black olives, pitted
- 1 tablespoon sesame paste

DIRECTIONS:

1. In a blender, mix the eggplant with salt, pepper the oil and the other ingredients, blend well and serve as a party spread.

Nutrition: *calories 215, fat 11, fiber 5.5, carbs 8, protein 7.6*

Preparation Time: 10 minutes
Cooking Time: 0 minutes
Servings: 6

203. Coconut Spread

INGREDIENTS:

- 2 garlic cloves, minced
- Juice of 1 lime
- 1 and ½ cups coconut cream
- 1 tablespoon Italian seasoning
- 4 spring onions, chopped
- A pinch of salt and black pepper
- 1 teaspoon oregano, dried
- 1 teaspoon mint, dried

DIRECTIONS:

1. In a blender, mix the coconut cream with the garlic, lime juice and the other ingredients, blend well and serve as a party spread.

Nutrition: *calories 210, fat 6.7, fiber 5.6, carbs 8, protein 5*

Preparation Time: 10 minutes
Cooking Time: 30 minutes
Servings: 4

204. Marinara Dip

INGREDIENTS:

- 2 garlic cloves, minced
- 1/2 cup water
- 32 oz. canned tomatoes, roughly chopped
- A pinch salt and black pepper
- 1/4 tsp. red pepper flakes, crushed

DIRECTION

1. In your instant pot, mix water with tomatoes, salt, pepper, pepper flakes and garlic.
2. Stir, cover and cook on High for 15 minutes.
3. Divide dip into small bowls and serve. Enjoy!

Nutrition: *Calories: 150 Cal Fat: 4 g Carbs: 21 g Protein: 10 g Fiber: 2 g*

CHAPTER 12: 21 DAY MEAL PLAN

DAYS	BREAKFAST	LUNCH/DINNER	DESSERT/SNACK
1	Cranberry Muffins	Spiced Okra	Green Bean Fries
2	Pineapple Oatmeal	Bell Peppers & Zucchini Stir Fry	Lemon Coconut Cilantro Rolls
3	Miso Oat Porridge	Spanish rice	Tamari Almonds
4	Mushroom Patties	Super tasty Vegetarian Chili	Spiced Popcorn
5	Peaches Oatmeal	Quinoa and Black Bean Lettuce Wraps	Mandarin Ambrosia
6	Poached Figs	Rice and Bean Lettuce Burgers	Coconut-Quinoa Pudding
7	Quinoa and Veggie Mix	Mexican Portobello Mushrooms	Stuffed Pears with Hazelnuts
8	Raspberry Curd	Potato Tempeh Hash	Buttermilk Panna Cotta with Mango
9	Rice Pudding	Vegan Spinach Pasta	Sweet Potato–Cinnamon Parfaits
10	Rice with Maple Syrup	White Couscous with Syrup	Sun-dried Tomato Pesto Snapper

DAYS	BREAKFAST	LUNCH/DINNER	DESSERT/SNACK
11	Strawberry Compote	Sautéed Collard Greens	Trout-Cilantro Packets
12	Turnip Dish	Creamy Chickpea Sandwiches	No Bake Mango Cheesecake
13	Spiced Sorghum & Berries	Flavorful Refried Beans	Vegan Mango Ice Cream with Brazil Nuts
14	Raw Cinnamon-Apple & Nut Bowl	Smoky Red Beans and Rice	Watermelon and Bell Pepper Slush
15	Peanut Butter & Cacao Breakfast Quinoa	Spicy Black-Eyed Peas	Blackberry Jam
16	Cauliflower Scramble	Coconut Mushroom Pizza	Kale Berry Delight
17	Veggie Breakfast Hash	Sweet Potato Chickpea Wraps	Veggie Cakes
18	Breakfast in Bangkok	Vegan Burgers	Cinnamon Coconut Chips
19	Chocolate and Banana Oatmeal	Black Bean Kale Salad Jars	Chocolate Brownies
20	French Toast with Berry Compote	Bulgur and Pinto Bean Lettuce Wraps	Rhubarb and Strawberry Dessert
21	Chocolate Chip and Coconut Pancakes	Barbecued Greens & Grits	Lemon Cake

CONCLUSION

Thank you for reading this book. The secret of the success of this type of diet is that it is a much healthier method for our body. But, also, it is a diet that is more respectful with the environment and that reduces our ecological impact. By basing the highest amount of plant intakes, you transform your diet into a more alkaline and physiological one, incorporating food-medicine within its many benefits:

Plants are high in fiber, which provides satiety, controls the absorption of glucose avoiding peaks of glycemia, stimulates the correct evacuation.

They have antioxidants, prevent premature aging, have anti-cancer and anti-inflammatory neuroprotective effects.

They are cleansing, they help eliminate toxins through our cleansing organs, liver, kidney, urine, fecal matter, perspiration.

They alkalize the body, which helps to compensate for acidosis caused by excess consumption of meat and/or processed foods.

Now that you have your own personal reasons for wanting to adopt a healthier diet and lifestyle, you have to power to move forward, and put action to your goals.

Adopting a whole foods, plant based diet, when paired with a reduction or elimination of animal products, can significantly reduce the amounts of saturated fats, and cholesterol that you consume. This has a dramatic effect on the way your body metabolizes food-especially fats. The fat already in your body gets trapped, because the food we consume usually has so much additional fat that our body must process the incoming foods before getting to our internal food storage. This turns into a cycle, because we are constantly consuming food that our body must find something to do with. The natural, short-term is to place the incoming fat into storage, in case we are ever starving in the future. Unfortunately, this is something that rarely comes in handy for those of us who never seem to be running on empty. The opportunity to use up our stored fat never arises because we just don't give it the chance.

In many cases, those who have adopted this lifestyle, and did it properly were able to lose a significant amount of weight over time. This is mostly because you are eating more vegetables and fruit (very dense in essential nutrients and low in calories), and avoiding foods that are high in calories and very low in nutrients, and disrupt the processes of digestion. Sticking to a whole food, plant based diet (when done properly) can bring about weight loss almost effortlessly. Sounds good to me!

Another one of the benefits of eating this particular diet is that you will be better able to control your insulin and glycemic levels. These two factors have an incredible impact on your health. They affect your hormones, your metabolism, and the levels of hunger that you experience.

The adoption of a plant based diet has been linked very closely with the clearing and strengthening of arterial walls. Real plant based foods can clear the built up plaque, and help to improve blood circulation. It is the only diet ever proven to reverse the #1 killer of men and women (heart disease) in the majority of patients.

Good luck.

Printed in Great Britain
by Amazon